I fucking love women. My love for women is the guiding force for everything I do. Women are my fucking muse, and I want to slowly contribute to a world in which we no longer feel we are fighting for space, but "lifting as we climb."

PRAISE FOR *WOMEN DON'T OWE YOU PRETTY*
BY FLORENCE GIVEN

-

"a fearless book"
Cosmopolitan

"an incredible mouthpiece for modern intersectional feminism"
Glamour

"game-changing"
Diva Magazine

"a vital read . . . empowering"
GayTimes

"rallying, radical, and pitched perfectly for her generation"
Evening Standard

"an accessible exploration of feminism built around the historic and modern expectations of women"
Living etc

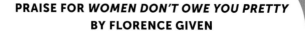

WRITTEN AND ILLUSTRATED BY

FLORENCE GIVEN

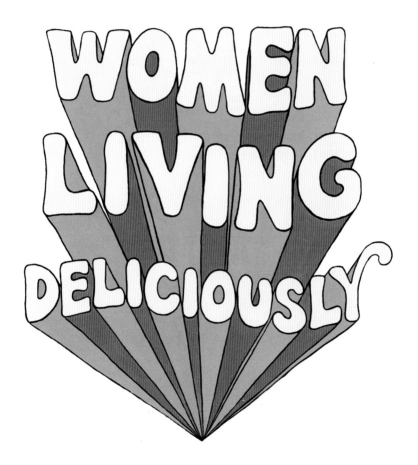

WOMEN LIVING DELICIOUSLY

SIMON ELEMENT

New York   London   Toronto   Sydney   New Delhi

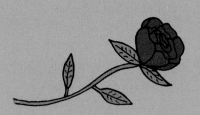

SIMON ELEMENT

An Imprint of Simon & Schuster, LLC
1230 Avenue of the Americas
New York, NY 10020

First Simon Element hardcover edition October 2024

SIMON ELEMENT is a trademark of Simon & Schuster, LLC

Simon & Schuster: Celebrating 100 Years of Publishing in 2024

For information about special discounts for bulk purchases, please contact Simon & Schuster Special Sales at 1-866-506-1949 or business@simonandschuster.com.

The Simon & Schuster Speakers Bureau can bring authors to your live event. For more information or to book an event, contact the Simon & Schuster Speakers Bureau at 1-866-248-3049 or visit our website at www.simonspeakers.com.

Interior design by Octopus Publishing Group

Manufactured in the United States of America

10 9 8 7 6 5 4 3

Library of Congress Cataloging-in-Publication Data has been applied for.

ISBN 978-1-6680-6712-3
ISBN 978-1-6680-6713-0 (ebook)

CONTENTS

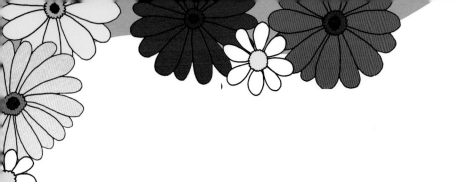

INTRODUCTION

I fucking love women.

I am aching to see a world full of women that love the shit out of their lives. Without apology, without disclaimers, without justifications. I am yearning to see a world in which women live fully in their bodies, using them the way they were intended: to experience, to relish, to cherish, and to enjoy every part of themselves. I want more women to discover the vibrant joy of living on their own terms. I want them to learn how to shine and become the sun in their own lives.

If you've picked up this book, I'm certain there's a part of you that knows you were meant for *more*. Part of you that's exhausted from a life of pleasing, shrinking, and striving to meet the expectations of others, desperate to expand and bloom beyond them. Part of you that craves connection with the more playful, alive, and carefree version of yourself behind the seriousness, stress, or resentment that can take over when life feels like *it's* running *you*. But that "spark" you're missing isn't within the pages of this book. It never left you to begin with. *She's still in there.* You just need to let her feel safe enough to come out.

You were not born to squeeze into the small roles written for you by others, but to take center fucking stage as the main character in your own life. You weren't born to be a human-sized Polly Pocket—pretty, perfect, static, and contained. To shrink, dim, and adjust yourself to make other people feel comfortable with your small existence. You were not put on this earth to make other people comfortable with the way you live, or for them to approve of the choices you make. A delicious life is not achieved through winning other people's approval of you, but through the courageous journey of discovering and embodying your *own* values, whether or not they're understood. If you don't design your life, it will be designed for you.

In my first book, *Women Don't Owe You Pretty*, I unpacked the ways that patriarchy has held women back for centuries and how it manifests in the world today. In this book, I am going to be shifting your attention towards the barriers society has created *within* you. I want to excavate the seeds of self-doubt that have grown like thick weeds in your mind, forming your entire fucking belief system. I want to unpack the way these beliefs have taken control of your life. And then I want you to expand *beyond* them. To unshackle yourself from the mental cages that have kept you living a fearful and much smaller life than the one you know you were meant for. I want this book to be a permission slip for you to courageously challenge the council of voices in your head that persuade you to minimize yourself. I want you to see that they have no real authority over your life when you decide to act against them. I want you to taste your full potential. You were meant for more and you fucking know it.

This is the book I wish that I could have handed to myself when I felt overwhelmed and numb to the beauty of life, to remind her that there is always something to live for, that no matter how stuck she feels, she always has the power to change *something*. To tell her that she doesn't need to shrink herself in fear of intimidating others and that it is safe for her to bloom. While these limits can be experienced in our minds, our outer experience of the world greatly affects those inner limits and how much we feel we are capable of—this will be harder for some people to challenge, depending on your identity, environment, and your responsibilities. Growth happens in baby steps and a beautiful life that invigorates you *does* exist—you just need a relentless belief that it is possible to achieve it. I hope to guide you into making more courageous decisions to stop pleasing others so that you, too, believe you're capable of creating a delicious life.

Although we cannot control what happens to us in life, we can control how we respond to it. We *can* control our next move. We each have the choice of what we do *with* the shit that's handed to us and I want nothing more than to remind you of your personal power and agency. Even if the only thing we have agency over is our perspective, through small actions we can begin to create real change in how we view ourselves: from feeling helplessly stuck in someone else's script to being an empowered individual capable of creating their own. Within our pain and trauma we can discover fertile soil for new beginnings.

I am writing this from my unique human perspective and, while I wouldn't dare attempt to encompass the entire collective female experience, I do hope that you can see parts of yourself in this book and my story—and that it leaves you feeling even a tiny bit more excited to be alive. While I also hope that one day we will be free from the limiting cage of gender roles, the terms "women" and "men" have been used throughout the book to simplify the ways that humans have all been socialized to fit ourselves within these binary roles. This is a book for anyone, regardless of your gender, who can relate to the nagging sense that you're getting in your own fucking way. Audacity is contagious and I hope some of mine rubs off on you.

I have split the book into three different stages. In the first part, **EXCAVATING: What's stealing your joy?**, we will expose the beliefs and habits that have been leeching and syphoning away your energy, so that you can call it back into yourself and intentionally redirect it into the things you fucking LOVE. What is holding you back? What voices lurk in your mind that keep you living small and fearfully? It may be uncomfortable at first, but we cannot change what we are not aware of.

The second part of the book, **PLANTING: Re-discovering you**, is all about how you can start to discover what the hell it is YOU truly want in life, so that you can begin to plant the seeds for the new ideas and beliefs you actually desire. This part of the book is the HOW on the road map for the ways you can implement more authenticity—and as a result more joy—into your life.

The third part of the book, **BLOOMING: Expanding into your delicious life**, is all action. You will no longer theorize the ways you can change your life or how you want to live it, but put it into courageous action, one step at a time. Your life will no longer take the shape of your fears, but slowly begin to reflect your desires as you allow your joy to become the new and rightful architect of it. This is about your season of blooming. This is where you reap the crops you have planted, relishing in the succulent fruits produced from your courage.

Women Living Deliciously was born because I wanted to exist in a world where a woman's value in society is not tied to how much of herself she's had to sacrifice for others. But one where she gets to do what sets her own soul on fire.

I want you to reach your full potential, to taste how delicious life can be. I want you to know with every fiber of your fucking being that it is not a selfish pursuit to love your life, but that it is generous—for feminism, for the world, for your family, for your career, for you—to live a life that brings you joy. The world needs more people who enjoy their lives.

So, let's begin with you.

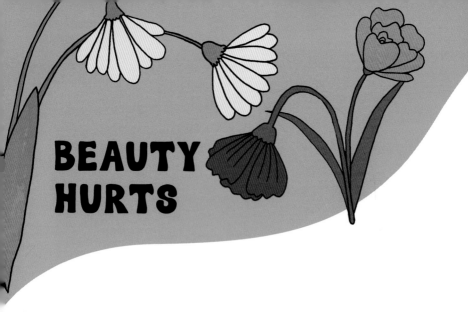

BEAUTY HURTS

"Your body is an instrument, not an ornament."
—Lindsay and Lexie Kite

Ever had a beautiful day out with your friends ruined by thinking about an "unflattering" picture someone took of you? Ever had incredible, delicious sex, only to be yanked out of the moment when you became conscious of your stomach rolls or cellulite? Ever wanted to look down at the person giving you head, but stopped as you imagined their view of your double chins? Breathed a sigh of relief when the person you're spooning with has fallen asleep, so you can finally relax and let go of your belly? Skipped a girls' holiday because the idea of being around other women's bodies makes you anxious? Been pulled out from a carefree state the second you walked into overhead lighting, afraid it would reveal the texture of your skin?

Women rarely get to fully and deliciously fucking RELAX. Our ability to enjoy our lives and "be in the moment" is constantly hindered and interrupted by an image-obsessed critical inner voice and the livestream it feeds us of our appearance. Rather than experiencing our lives through our bodies in the here and now, our attention is often absorbed by the thoughts in our heads. It is so hard for us to exist FULLY inside our own bodies when we are taught to constantly observe them. We are unable to "sink into the moment" because we cannot escape our self-conscious thoughts.

How much more energy will we waste in this precious life on the imagined judgments of others? How much more energy will we waste on monitoring our appearance when we could be spending our time living, creating, dancing, relishing, and being fully present? What kind of a world would be created if women unshackled the mental resources spent on perfecting themselves? Where would that energy go, what beautiful things would it produce in the world?

Renee Engeln calls this cultural obsession Beauty Sickness, defining it as "what happens when women's emotional energy gets so bound up with what they see in the mirror that it becomes harder for them to see other aspects of their lives." There have been *plenty* of times when I have "called in Beauty Sick." Canceled plans. Not shown up *purely* because the stress of being pretty had become all consuming. Most of us can remember a time when we skipped attending something because we didn't feel we looked good enough to be there. Because we didn't feel perfect or pretty enough to live our own *fucking* lives! Beauty Sickness reminds me of the days on the beach I missed, the sex I couldn't bring myself to enjoy *because if I can't even look at my body, why would anyone else want to?*, all the swims I never went for in the sea, the clothes I wouldn't wear out of shame, or the food I wouldn't "allow myself" to eat during family holidays or group dinners. I lived in a normalized, constant denial of any experience of joy or pleasure, to please others and project an image of perfection, constantly making myself smaller, or even invisible by not attending altogether. Even with the events that I did attend, there were too many times I was physically present, but mentally vacant—as a hefty chunk of my attention was focused on how I looked. If I'd had to be brutally honest and write down the real reason for my lack of attendance on RSVP slips, most of them would have said, *"Can't come, not feeling pretty enough, throwing my clothes all over the room, screaming, crying in the mirror. Have overwhelming anxiety about the dress code, am afraid no one there will like me, that I won't be good enough."* The worst part is that we grow up to think this is a normal part of being a girl. But existing is not supposed to be this stressful.

In case you're thinking, *We're past all that shit now,* we

really, really aren't. If your own experience of having entire days ruined because you didn't think you looked pretty isn't enough proof, Renee Engeln cites the depressing statistic that 34 percent of girls aged five (yes, fucking five-year-olds!) report restricting their diet at least "sometimes." Young girls learn to create boundaries with food before they learn how to have boundaries with other people. The separation of a woman from her own body starts so young.

The distorted thoughts we have about ourselves when eating, dressing up, and looking in the mirror are not the "truth"—they are a habit. They are messages that have been implanted into our minds, messages that have been absorbed from our environment. They are our programming. We receive nudges and social cues throughout our lives which push us to feel we are not worthy of living until we are perfect. Perhaps it was the cruel objectifying headline you read about a woman's beach body on the magazine cover your mom left on the table. The way you watched the girls around you discuss their figures at school. How they sucked in their stomachs to "not look pregnant," which led you to buy the stomach-shrinking lingerie you found next to the aisle of bras. How the girls around you started to order less food at lunch with the phrase, "No bread for me, I'm being good!" Wanting to fit in you thought, *Perhaps I should do the same, I want to be good!* When these thoughts are left unchecked and accepted passively they seed themselves in the soil of our minds and begin to grow and root, becoming thick, stubborn beliefs we later realize in adulthood we did not choose.

When we don't interrogate these weed-like thoughts, they grow deeper, thicker, and stronger. We start to say it's just "who we are." No longer something we have merely overheard, they become deeply accepted, rooted, and nurtured in our minds as our beliefs. This outside voice we hear from others becomes the inner abusive voice we use to talk to ourselves. Yes. It is abusive. How would it make you feel to say out loud to another person the things you tolerate from within? *"I can't even look at you in the mirror today, you're disgusting." "No one would want to look at you, hide yourself." "How is anyone ever going to love you?" "You're a failure who doesn't deserve anything."* It hurts me to even write these things down and to publish them in a book! Just as you would defend your friend from someone who was saying these things, you must defend yourself from the voice that reverberates in your mind. You must cultivate *another, kinder* voice, a separate one that talks *back* to the critical one in your head. Otherwise, you become your worst critic. You mistake it for who you are.

In a world where we have culturally pressured and convinced women to obsess over every inch of their bodies and pull them apart, it makes you wonder . . . *was this the plan all along—to intentionally exhaust us? To drain us of our source of power? To create obstacles in our path that make it harder to think and feel clearly?*

Years ago, I was running late to a therapy session in the middle of a hot London summer. I was wearing a tight pair of cycling shorts, a bra, and a blazer. On my commute I was experiencing severe anxiety and struggling to take in a full breath. I had to keep yawning in order to take in oxygen fully. I brushed it off and thought to myself, *This just happens when I wear tight clothes.* Once I arrived at my therapist's office I told her about my erratic breathing. She asked me when it started. I thought back to a date around two weeks earlier. She nodded slowly, pursing her lips. "Wasn't that when that man made those rude comments about the shape of your stomach?" I nodded—"I think so, why?" As soon as the words fell out of my mouth, it clicked. "I think you've been subconsciously sucking in your stomach since you read those comments, I think it's restricting your breathing. You're taking shallow breaths which is triggering anxiety." Even as she said these words, I was clenching in my stomach. I took a deep inhale and, on the exhale, my stomach stretched the tight shorts to their fullest and I'd taken a deep breath for the first time in weeks. Well fuck. She was right. The worst part is that I didn't even know I was doing it! Those words about my body from that man had been passively accepted by my mind without me knowing, adding fertilizer to the overgrowth already there. By sucking in my stomach, my brain was trying to protect the part of me that had been "attacked." This all happened without my awareness. Frightening fucking stuff! Beauty Sickness has a lot of us witnessing our bodies instead of existing in them fully, even to the detriment of our own comfort. I have spent years watching my body twice. Once through my own eyes, the other through the imagined gaze of others.

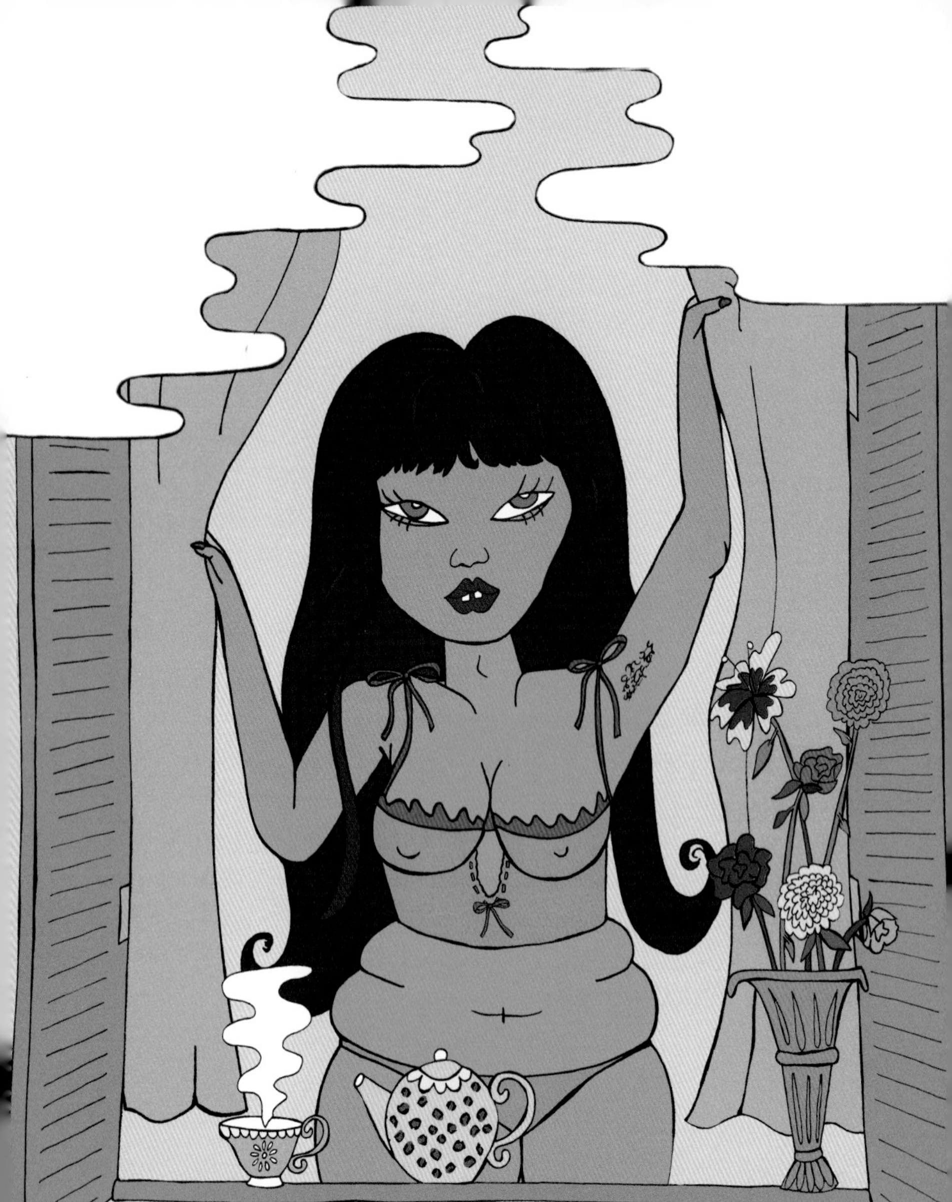

MY BODY IS A BEAUTIFUL VESSEL THAT EXISTS FOR ME TO EXPERIENCE LIFE!

I once found myself sucking in my stomach reflexively when a man looked in my direction on the set of a photo shoot. As though I'd been caught off guard by literally *breathing*, like a woman who'd gone off-script, and had to quickly pull herself back into perfect composure to "step into her role." *Why* did I do this, when I know I am *not* a doll, or an object, but a breathing woman with a stomach full of life? I felt the second round of *feminist* shame, for realizing how instinctual it was. He didn't force me to suck in my stomach. He just looked at me. Yet something inside me "knew" to do it. Isn't that frightening? The way we learn to bend and contort our entire existence into something presentably doll-like at the expense of our comfort and health. It is not our fault, it is a habit we have been beguilingly encouraged to adopt, to slow us down and drain us.

THE OBJECTIFIED

If you look around you, you will see some objects—your phone, a cup, a pen, this book. Do any of these things have a life or an existence outside your use for them? No, of course not, they are objects! They cannot feel. They are things you bought, only of use and with value when you decide to use them, or when you have deemed them worthy enough of having on display. An object is *experienced* by something or someone else. An object exists for the visual, sensual, functional, inspirational purposes of somebody. It does not have a say in how it is used. It is "ornamental."

Women have long been objectified in this same way under patriarchy. Women have been treated as though we are objects, beings that are decorative and functional, no different from the book, the cup, the vase of flowers. We exist for the visual pleasure of the people around us who are given permission to experience us—men. We have internalized this belief and it has resulted in the *self*-objectification of our own bodies. We do not need to receive a reminder to be beautiful, this obligation is carried with us into the privacy of our bedrooms, every time we catch our reflection in a mirror, every time we walk past the eyes of a human being, pulling us out of the present moment. We are unable to fully experience our lives but instead *watch* ourselves experiencing our lives, through the eyes of the person experiencing us.

According to John Berger, "Men look at women. Women watch themselves being looked at. This determines not only most relations between men and women, but also the relation of women to themselves. The surveyor of a woman in herself is male: the surveyed female. Thus she turns herself into an object—and most particularly an object of vision: a sight."

An object cannot experience. Objects *are experienced*. No wonder we are still so horrified when women have opinions—objects aren't supposed to talk back, *they're inanimate*.

Think of a summer day at the beach. If you believed yourself to be a human being—here to *experience*—the way your body looked would not be an issue. It would not be the focal point of your entire day, perhaps even preventing you from going in the sea. The objectification of our bodies prevents us relishing life because on some level, we believe we are ornamental. But we are not objects, we are human fucking beings who deserve to experience. To feel the salty water and the hard grains of sand between our toes. That is what our senses are for and that is what we will miss when we die, when we no longer have the *privilege* of a body. The world we live in is unfair—people treat us according to our appearance—and guess fucking what? We cannot let that stop us from living our lives. We can listen to that fucking voice in our heads telling us to stay at home, telling us we need to order a whole new outfit before a trip to the beach, that we're not good looking enough—and we can fucking ignore it. We can go as we are. We deserve to participate in our own lives.

The only way to no longer be a victim of this training is to disobey it. How our bodies look shouldn't control how we live and experience our lives, yet it does. Every day. This disconnect from our humanity has devastating effects on our ability to live life. Women and young girls have been robbed for so long of the mindset of a full human being who exists to experience. We have slowly withdrawn ourselves from life's pleasures until we are deemed physically beautiful enough to jump in and participate.

Since an object cannot feel, the transition out of self-objectification lies in pursuing pleasure and experiences of FEELING. It lies in creating a world that delights us to transition from viewing our bodies as something to be looked at (an object), into something to be lived in (a person having an experience). The path out of self-objectification is to experience and feel things with our bodies, gently bringing our attention back to the present moment. With each step we tell our subconscious that we exist to LIVE!

A person never looks more beautiful than when they are doing something they love. When, for just a second, I catch a woman off guard—passionately expressing herself, laughing, dancing, forgetting how she looks—it is a glow like no other, an inside-out radiance, a beauty that shines from within. The kind of embodied beauty that does not come from controlling her image, but an immersive beauty in an experience that demands all her attention. Yet we have been taught to fear losing control over our image, shutting off the self-surveillance, because we do not think that we will be beautiful without it. We think people will be horrified by what they see. By who we are.

In the media, we read headlines about women who dare to leave their home with messy hair. They say, "Uh-oh! She's let herself go!" as though that's a bad thing. As though letting go of a fixation on image *isn't* the path to a happy life. GOOD FOR HER! Women are so beautiful when we let ourselves go. When we dare to give so much attention to something that we forget what we look like! When we prioritize the experience we are having over how we look while we experience it. We may not feel "pretty" when we "let ourselves go"—whether concentrating, working, walking, fucking and moaning and scrunching up our faces the way we want—but we will FEEL damn good.

And the irony is that when women *feel* good, we emanate an astronomical beauty, a glow from within, that is far more powerful than any external tools we might use to impress others with our beauty. Because this kind of beauty cannot be touched. It cannot be taken. It's an internal light switch only we can access, using the things we love in our lives to turn ourselves the fuck on.

BEAUTY IMPULSE

I notice when a woman momentarily objectifies herself. I can spot it because I recognize it in myself. A glaze rolls over her eyes when someone walks past, a quick head jerk to her "photogenic" side, a clenching in of her stomach, a covering up of a blemish on her face with her hand, a lifting of her head during sex to avoid "multiple chins" because she dared to lose herself to full bodily pleasure. It's like a fidgety beauty impulse! Always camera ready, but there are no cameras except the one in her mind, living under the male gaze microscope and believing she is always a slip-up away from magnifying her flaws. I am still unlearning this shit myself. This process of becoming an object of "sight," as John Berger describes, has become our instinctual autopilot.

How are we ever supposed to sink fully into the delicious "now" if even our breathing is being subconsciously restricted, stomachs clenched and monitored? How are we ever supposed to feel the joy of having a body, when all we see when we look into the eyes of another person are all the flaws and imperfections we clocked in the mirror on our way out of the house? Preempting someone's judgment of us by excusing ourselves with, "Ah I look like such a mess ...!"?

Well, *it's literally fucking impossible.*

Beauty standards were invented to drain us.

You know those energy-efficiency ratings you can get for your home? If there was an energy-efficiency rating that could describe you as a person, what would it say? How much energy is being siphoned out of you, lost to rumination, doing things you don't want to out of a need to please, or focusing on your appearance? Imagine where that energy could go if you patched the holes up and directed all of that energy back into what brings you joy instead....

Often, we don't even know that we're doing it. Women have been taught that the best place to invest their energy is on caring about and safeguarding their looks to the degree that at times it is the sole focus of our lives. We must pluck any wayward hairs. Put on our "face." Spend ages in front of the mirror making it look like we just woke up like this. Plan our outfits to be the perfect balance of a little bit desirable, but never too desirable so we are not followed home. Bring an extra layer of clothing for safety on the journey home. Find a bag big enough for our belongings because none of our actual clothes have pockets in them. Leave a hallway light on. Pack extra makeup so our faces are constantly perfectible. Leaving home for women is an elaborate fucking art form. Men cannot comprehend the invisible and intentional decision-making process that goes into a woman simply trying to leave the bloody house! When all a man has to do is to be clean and brush his teeth, maybe smell good. At a push. In a world where we do not feel safe to relax in public, leaving home is a rigorous process of managing as much of our appearance as we possibly can for a false sense of control. Beauty rituals and "putting on her face" often feel as though they are a woman's defense mechanism before she steps out into the world, her protective shield to fight off unwanted remarks and stares that remind her of how she looks in every glance. In the words of John Berger, "Women constantly meet glances which act like mirrors, reminding them of how they look or how they should look. Behind every glance there is judgment."

We would simply be too powerful if this energy was invested into our actual lives. The more women have gained social freedom, the more a distraction had to be created. Otherwise, we might realize our partners don't treat us well. We might have more time to excel over men in the workforce. More confidence to contribute in meetings. Beauty Sickness slows us down and that is not an accident, it's an intentional design. Writing back in the nineties, Naomi Wolf was audaciously blunt about this, saying, "Beauty discrimination (in the workplace) has become necessary, not from the perception that women will not be good enough, but that they will be, as they have been, twice as good." In *The Beauty Myth* she details the entire history of women as hardworking people. When women started to enter the (paid) workforce, employers had essentially hired people who had already been working hard, for free, in the domestic sphere. Because this wasn't valued as "real work" no one saw the threat coming when we entered the workplace. "Women work hard—twice as hard as men. All over the world, and for longer than records have been kept, that has been true." A distraction had to be created. Fast.

Because if women's attention is focused on our looks, you can guarantee our insecurities and self-conscious thoughts will magnify day by day, clouding the prime real estate of our minds so that we don't have the energy to pay attention to anything else. Certainly not enough energy to fight upstream and change these systems. The less embodied and whole we are—the more fragmented and self-conscious our attention is, seeing ourselves as parts that need to be fixed, decorative beings to be looked at and not living breathing creatures—the easier it is to control us.

We busy women's precious resource of energy with the false promise that the more beautiful we are and the more time we focus on our beauty, the more we will be fulfilled and able to achieve the same power as men. This lie had all of us fooled into thinking that starving ourselves every day to be skinnier, and spending money on products to waste our financial resources, was not only empowering, but a worthwhile pursuit of happiness. But the privileges of this "beauty" standard fade as we grow older, when we're deemed "past our shelf life," when we realize half of our lives have been spent not being present but pursuing something that was fucking quicksand. Who do we blame for these feelings when this natural, aging process happens? Patriarchy? No! We blame ourselves, the way we're trained to. We are geared to turn towards self-improvement. Creams. Diets. Surgeries. We think it's our own fault for getting so "unattractive" and "old." Loving ourselves is not a good business plan for capitalism. Capitalism *relies* on our self-hatred to exist.

We are taught to outsource our worth to other people. In the words of Naomi Wolf, "Women's identity must be premised upon 'beauty' so that we will remain vulnerable to outside approval, carrying the vital sensitive organ of self-esteem exposed to the air." When we stop to consider how much of our lives and energy we're leaking out to the exhausting and futile pursuit of perfection, it becomes alarmingly clear that this is no mistake. Most of us would not *choose* to live our lives in this way if there were no consequences for not conforming. Girls are not inherently beauty-obsessed, they are trained to be.

So when we consider that these habits are not "natural," but built over time, developed throughout our lives as smart solutions to our problems, we can start to realize that there are many things in our lives that we are not actively and consciously choosing for ourselves, but defaulting to. The habits were not planted and seeded by us, but by others—accepted into the soil of our minds to grow and take over our plots. They were not created in response to our individual authentic desires, but in reaction to an environment that needs insecure women and consumers. How many of the things we do come from a place of fear instead of joy?

In this book, I want to draw your attention to how our perfection-obsessed culture and our fixation on moral purity as a pillar of womanhood, is preventing us from experiencing joy and appreciating what is beautiful in our lives_paying attention to the things that don't need changing or fixing, but are beautiful and wholly ours for the relishing! It is no mistake that we may feel "guilty" for enjoying our lives, or daring to want more. To feel "enough" means we might slow down and realize there's a bunch of shit we were buying, people we were dating, thoughts we were endorsing, that we didn't need after all. We may discover we are enough without them!

I'm almost certain that on my death bed I will not be lamenting the size of my stomach, my thighs, or how many good skin days I had over my lifetime, but instead how many of those days of life I missed out on because the warped view of my body stopped me from living the fullest, most expansive version of my life possible. I don't want any of us to realize too late that we have been living a small and joy-restricted diet-version of what our lives could be, because we were waiting to be perfect enough to enjoy ourselves. Our lives should be fat and full of EVERYTHING.

BAIT-AND-SWITCH

Though women have gained a lot of rights to our bodies and it is not "as bad as it used to be," the control that government and corporations have over our bodies hasn't actually gone anywhere. It has just evolved. Naomi Wolf explains that after the 1970s when women finally gained more legal and social freedoms in the form of birth control, reproductive rights, and credit cards and were considered to have properly entered the workplace, a much stealthier form of control had to be developed as a counterattack to these newfound freedoms. A woman would no longer be told directly what to do, but would be coerced through advertising and an oversaturation of images of the "ideal" woman, into controlling, dieting, and restricting *herself*. The best part? She would buy the makeup brush, the razor, and the diet pills with her own money, and think it was her own empowering choice. It's pretty fucking clever, since it now has women controlling and regulating their own bodies. The government no longer has to intervene, women are "voluntarily" doing it to themselves. In a culture that has deliberately set the standards of women's beauty so high that they are unachievable and force us all to comply *or else*, how can we tell if it's a choice, when femininity is forced onto us from a young age? When a beauty decision is framed persuasively as "self-improvement" it can be hard to resist buying into it. *We're supposed to want to be the best version of ourselves, right?* Especially if it's what our friends are doing. Especially if it's what everyone on social media is doing. Especially if it makes us *pretty.*

When you start to discuss feminism with someone who believes women are now totally equal to men, most will innocently point to all the progress women have made. If it's a man saying this—which it usually is—he might even point to *you* and say, "You make more money than *me*!" as some sort of proof that sexism does not exist anymore. You try to explain the gender pay gap to him and he might say, "Women just don't ask for raises!" This reply might even leave *you* feeling silly. *What can you say back to that?! He's right!* You might feel embarrassed at your inability to explain to someone how women are still controlled by patriarchy, fumbling over your words as you can't find the arguments to counter the apparent facts and logic. But that's because even though the cage that prevents women from rising is no longer so flagrantly placed around us in the form of laws and legislation, the patriarchal cage that controls women is still inside our own fucking *minds.*

There is still another obstacle to fight, and it is inside us.

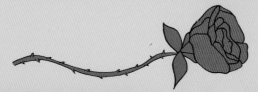

BREAKING UP WITH THE PATRIARCHY

The aim is to control women. It always has been.

Women are collectively breaking up with the patriarchy, as we slowly awaken to the way it has tricked us into living small and fearful lives by penetrating our minds. Much like trying to exit a narcissistic relationship with a toxic partner, it's messy, they play dirty, they pull out their worst tricks before they eventually lose their control over you. This is what we are seeing today. Now that we are more mentally free and beginning to wake up, the patriarchy and governing bodies can sense this. They know that *we* know. So as women become wise to their controlling tactics, the patriarchy restructures the game to develop stealthier tactics and maintain power, while giving the illusion that it is over. Naomi Wolf says this is like an "adult, play wrestling a child, enjoying letting the child feel it has won." It doesn't strike me as a coincidence that the rise in body positivity and women having increasing agency over their bodies has been met with a counterattack to regress reproductive rights in the US, reversing the *Roe v Wade* decision to allow abortions. As the world moves on from the suffocating expectations placed on the roles of "man" and "woman" and there is more room to be who we want to be, we see that the rights of trans people are being used as a battleground for people to play out their frustration, to defend what's left of their sense of identity as they watch the roles that have defined them their whole lives crumble before their eyes, and attack the people who have the courage to challenge the gender roles they were assigned, and say, "I am neither a man nor a woman."

Breaking up with patriarchy and the ways it has formed within our minds will not be smooth. When access to reproductive rights was expanded, it was a bait-and-switch. We thought we were getting freedom, but the cage became internal. Now that we have started to suss this out, the legislation is creeping up on us again. Control over women never stopped. Patriarchy is like a toxic boyfriend—once you call out his controlling behavior, he promises to start seeing a therapist. He goes to see the therapist, learns a bunch of therapy jargon, and his abuse becomes more covert, less traceable. Maybe he starts passively controlling the way you dress by not giving you as much affection when you wear certain clothing or by comparing you to other women. You now learn to associate the clothes you want to wear with uncomfortable feelings and a lack of affection. So you decide not to wear that dress anymore. *Why not, if it makes him happy? Plus, he didn't tell me not to wear it! This is my choice!* It may seem like a "choice," you might even convince yourself that you don't like the clothes anymore, or that "doing some things to please your partner is normal," but it's a result of his desire to stop you wearing them. His methods have just become smarter. He has now found out how to manipulate you into doing something he desires without getting his hands dirty. He has got you to mistrust your intuition and give him what he wants. This is the same way patriarchy has got what it wants, a slowing down of the progress of women financially, sexually, and mentally with the illusion that we are "choosing" this image-obsessed path ourselves. It is horrendous that we have the audacity to call some women "self-obsessed" as an insult, as though it is a personal flaw and not a habit of survival they have developed in a culture that demands perfection.

Beauty as a form of control was introduced to destabilize a woman's self-esteem. Not only does the obsession with beauty distract us from what's important, the hunger and starvation we put ourselves through from diet culture weakens our bodies. We miss out on so much of our lives because we're not really there. We're watching ourselves instead—voyeurs of our own existence. We might order a side dish when we want to have the same meal as everyone else. We go to events burdened with the paranoia of being photographed from our bad side like it's the literal dark side of the bloody moon, hiding the differences in our bodies compared to others. The most important days and beautiful moments of our lives are often completely overwhelmed by our tsunami of concern and fear about how we look. Our obsession with our image impacts our ability to be present, the ability to live fully in our bodies and soak up the richness of our everyday lives. How are we supposed to soak up the beauty of a sunset on the beach when our attention is focused on how our stomachs look over the top of our bikini bottoms? Or the hair we forgot to shave on our toes? There is no way for the love that life is trying to offer us to get in, for the joy to pour out, it is being blocked.

When we do not feel enough, we never consider whether it is the *lens* we are viewing ourselves through that's broken, not ourselves. We have been socialized in such a way that we have no problem apologizing for and assuming— if not all—most of the blame in any situation. Think back to a time when you hid something from your friend about someone you were dating, so they wouldn't hate that person. Or dismissed someone's poor treatment of you and explained it away with, "It's probably because of their past" so *they* didn't feel uncomfortable about what *they* did to you. Most of us are taught to be "nice girls." And nice girls don't make people uncomfortable. They make everyone feel fucking great about themselves! So we learn to absorb responsibility for things that are not our responsibility, to save people from facing the consequences of their own actions. This cultural guilt and knee-jerk reaction to absorb blame sets us up to assume the fault is with *us* at every turn. It convinces us we need fixing. We are trained to see ourselves as at fault and buy into self-improvement and bodily restriction. We assume the blame and take accountability for our "flaws."

While it's easy to view this realization as depressing, I promise it will eventually be empowering. Because now we can begin the courageous journey of redirecting our energy! Calling it back from the places we have unconsciously invested it, that are giving us no return, to instead begin placing it into the things that reward

and fulfil us. It is a
lifelong process but it will
be worth it. You're quite literally going
to feel the energy pouring back into your life,
invigorating everything within you and around you.
One boundary set, one earlier night, one cruel beauty expectation lowered for yourself at a time.

This awareness allows you to start asking yourself questions
about where your energy goes, such as, *Why does getting dressed always
make me feel crap?* It might be because you believed you needed to prove
yourself with every outfit. You realize you're exhausted, because you over-
commit to social events in fear of being seen as unfriendly, when you would
rather stay at home. You realize you never liked wearing dresses and ignored
your body's way of telling you this, because you inherited the belief that
"beauty is pain."

It's so fucking powerful taking even the slowest of steps towards a life that
will leave you feeling deliciously satisfied, instead of resentful, exhausted,
and starving for more. There are as many ways to feel resentful and exhausted
as there are people in the world; for me it was because I was constantly trying
to live up to someone else's standard of *good enough*. Instead, though, we can
all inch closer towards a life lived according to the values of our own choosing,
as we weed out old beliefs and decide to plant the seeds for what we want to
come to fruition in our life next. Whatever you wish. You can grow it. A life
of your design, not of default. I'm not saying it's easy, you will have to sacrifice
something. But part of you already knew that. Often, that's the reason we
avoid change in the first place. We're afraid of what we will lose. If we relin-
quish our tight grasp on beauty rituals, some might say we've "let ourselves
go." When we set boundaries, some people might not like the fact they can't
have as much access to us anymore and leave. But what we "lose" in reputation
with others, we gain in respect for *ourselves*. Making choices aligned to our
values instead is a bold and courageous move. It's delicious as fuck!

Chasing perfection in every area of our lives will forever leave us unsatisfied, because it does not exist. As long as we still believe that "perfect" exists and we measure ourselves against this patriarchal simulation, we will always come up short. We will never be happy. It will never be enough. In a world where a literal fucking *body shape* can go out of fashion, nothing we do will ever satiate the hunger for perfection inside ourselves, as tomorrow, our body shape could be deemed "worthless" by some trend forecaster. Perfect does not exist.

Because a lot of our energy is being spent on our beauty, measuring and comparing it against others, we can become numb to the sheer abundance and beauty in both ourselves and the world around us. All we have been trained to spot is *lack*. We have minds trained to spot what *isn't* there, as opposed to what *is*, to keep us reaching, proving, spending, perfecting. This is one of the reasons we are often dissatisfied, even after getting something we want. We return to our default state of "wanting," once again. Obsession with achieving perfection in any form removes us from a state of gratitude and of appreciating what we have.

Wouldn't it be pretty dull if the purpose of our lives was to suffer on our way to becoming as skinny and perfect as possible? Do you really think that's what mother nature intended for each of us? Of course fucking not! Just look at everything we were given. Bright succulent fruits growing on trees, ready to pick and gorge on. A sun that does not stop shining, sustaining and giving life and joy to everything it touches. The many forms of love we can feel from other human beings. The euphoric bliss of a good album. A tongue to taste everything with. I was literally born with a clitoris, for fuck's sake. Pleasure was not the afterthought of whatever created us, *but part of the design!* Everything I have been taught about my body in the world has gone against the truth and the nature of what my body is here to actually do. Our bodies are here to *experience.* Instead, we have trained women, who were born to relish in the privilege of having a body, to police it, controlling and punishing it for "bad behavior." In the diet program Slimming World, certain foods are actually called "syns" (I'm sure the pun is lost on no one). *Doesn't this word choice say everything about the moral perfectionism we assign to every choice we make?*

Breaking up with patriarchy is, by extension, a form of breaking up with ourselves, since the patriarchy's structure has formed inside our minds and we have falsely identified with these beliefs as "who we are" for so long. Much of it has formed our personalities! To experience the joy we desire, for us to get to the end of our lives and feel we have lived them fully, we need to first begin by identifying the beliefs that have been planted in our minds, so that we can overcome the limits they have created and expand BEYOND them.

We need to talk about the ways women have been trained to keep ourselves SMALL and to fear our own expansion. Brief warning: it might piss you off.

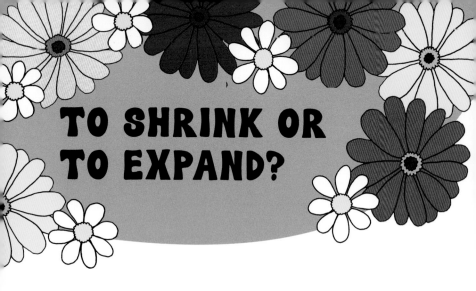

TO SHRINK OR TO EXPAND?

We know that we often create limits for ourselves in our minds about what we think we're capable of achieving, due to a lack of self-belief. But there's another limit we have: how much we *want* to achieve. How much we *want* to be happy. Subconsciously, we may even fear success! In the words of Jo Freeman, author of *Trashing: The Dark Side of Sisterhood*, "Women exhibiting potential for achievement are punished by both women and men. The 'fear of success' is quite rational when one knows that the consequence of achievement is hostility and not praise." Even if we say we want to be very successful, as long as part of us secretly fears success, happiness, joy, or shining "too bright," it will be driving our behavior and sabotaging our chances of achieving this. We need to discuss how women have learned to make themselves smaller and shrink—to avoid exhibiting "too much" excellence and being punished for it. To avoid committing what Gay Hendricks calls "*the crime of outshining.*"

There are two opposing truths that women must straddle:

1. If we are going to live our best lives and be joyful on our own terms, we must "EXPAND." We must take risks, we must learn to use the word "NO," we must leave our comfort zones, leave our homes to experience life, try new things, enter fresh and unknown territory, push through the limiting beliefs we have inherited that tell us the way we are is bad. We must travel, share our thoughts with others, express ourselves, assert ourselves, speak our minds, learn to choose what's right for us even if it means disappointing the people who love us.

2. Every step of the way, something inside us will kick in and make us want to "SHRINK." If we try any of these things, we place ourselves in the path of criticism, envy, jealousy, attacks, harassment, social isolation, bullying, and people not liking us. No matter how much we say we want to live a delicious life, our brains—wired to protect us—will step in and convince us to SHRINK.

When we have watched every successful woman be torn to shreds, when every other night there is a new story of a woman being stalked and followed home, is it any wonder so many women live fearful, small lives? As a woman grows into herself, she becomes torn between honoring her desire to bloom and expand, and honoring her survival instinct to shrink and play it small. More often than not, we don't think we have a choice and default to the latter. Let's step into the entangled world of joy and feminism.

To be carefree, we need to first address the "phantom" structure that cages us all. How the fuck do we start to "live deliciously," when our brains are trained to keep us safe from harm and our experience as women teaches us to believe there is harm coming for us everywhere? We know and have heard a million times over that the only way to experience happiness is to remain "open" to life, and yet it is when we were open to life that we experienced some of the most traumatic events. We watch women be harassed for wearing certain clothes, slandered publicly for expressing themselves, their bodies debated in group chats and magazine headlines, sexually assaulted after meeting someone from a dating app, excluded from friendship groups for growing. We know that outside our comfort zone is where life begins, yet women learn—not through mind-manufactured fear but through lived experience—that to cross that line is a threat to our safety. Why on earth would you *WANT* that?

But here's the thing. I have tried living like that. I have tried being small. Wearing less color. Not leaving the house. Not going on dates. And guess what? Nothing fucking happened. No joy, no connection, no self-development, no lessons, no laughter, no life. If we shrink in response to our fear all the time, our pain still controls our lives. The danger can be very, very real. The world *can* be scary. Men *can* be terrifying. Women *can* be mean. But we cannot, under any fucking circumstances, allow fear to stop us from living our lives and becoming open to life and love again. We cannot allow the selfish actions of others to terrify us away from the delicious, fat, juicy life we deserve, the life that will bring us love and joy. We cannot allow the fear instilled in us by patriarchy to keep us living small, self-protective lives.

CONDITIONED FOR SMALLNESS

So, why *is* "small" the default for women?

The world has to try so fucking hard to convince women to be small, because we are *not* fucking small. If we were, we would not need convincing.

We are coerced into "small" everything. Small waist. Small thighs. Small ambition. Small desires. Small passion. Small intellect. Small needs. Small feelings. Some women submit to the rules of this smallness, only to realize they have swung the pendulum too far and need to start asserting themselves to live a life on their own terms. Not all women conform, of course. There are some women who actively rebel against "small," only to realize later through suffering and burnout that they have swung the pendulum too far in the opposite direction. Most of us have experienced our fair share of both. I am a woman with ambition bigger than my human limits who goes for every single thing she fucking wants, but also a woman who is still learning to set her boundaries. And truthfully, rebelling against our cultural conditioning is just as exhausting as submitting to it. The work is about finding our equilibrium, trying to balance these two polarizing energies within us. Rejecting neither our desire for expansion, nor our survival need to shrink. Fear serves its purpose. But it's about fine-tuning our intuition to detect when the threat is real, and when it's that fearful voice preventing us from doing something exciting. When we can honor both these parts we become whole and integrated.

We learn our "place" in the world early on. We learn that to threaten the social contract of what a woman "should" be by daring to be our full, authentic, and lively selves is a social death that could risk isolation, and so we learn to stay small. But there are parts of us that want to bloom. Desire leadership.

Desire expression. Dreams we have. FUCKS to give! So we constantly wrestle with these two conflicting instincts: to express ourselves and be seen by others and the part of ourselves that is afraid of how we'll be treated. To shrink, or to expand?

To shrink in the face of fear is nothing to be ashamed of. Fear is a smart instinct we have learned to keep us safe from danger; both our brains and bodies use it to protect us. But it means we have brains wired for surviving, not thriving. I need you to really understand this: your brain is not wired for joy, it is wired for *survival*. Which is a good thing for your safety, but an absolute shit show for your happiness! If you want to be happy, it means that you are going to have to actively seek out joy while *ignoring* that voice of fear in your head, because it isn't fucking going anywhere. It is literally BUILT IN there. If you're a woman who has been raised to be good and pure, even betraying the voice in your head can make you feel bad. This fearful voice is like an over-protective parent who loves you so much that they want to keep you out of any possible danger or rejection. But being wrapped in protection doesn't allow you to make mistakes, learn or build a sense of who you are and what you are capable of. That fearful voice is going to tell you not to go to the beach, *because what if people don't like your body?* That fearful voice is going to tell you not to go on that date, *because what if they break your heart and reject you?* By stopping you from doing scary things, the voice doesn't let you learn for yourself that you're far more capable than you think; that if you do go to the beach, sure, you might find that you're nervous at first on the car ride there, but that your worries will shrink within seconds of hearing the laughter and giddiness of your friends, allowing you to relax and experience the healing power of the sun and ocean on your skin. Or that you will survive the nerves of the date it's telling you not to go on, because they end up being hilarious and you diffuse the nerves through laughter, and get to feel the enticing charge of attraction with a sexy stranger.

Fear is not a good teacher; it prevents us from self-discovery. It stops us from learning that we are capable of handling uncertainty in life, that we can learn to dance with it. Listening

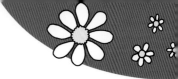

to this voice is what holds us back from living a life on our own terms. It stops us from fine-tuning our connection to our intuition, by robbing us of the life experiences required for discerning what it even sounds and feels like! For example, I didn't know that feeling nauseous and having heart palpitations after a first date walked through the door and hugged me was a "red flag" and not just "butterflies," until I compared it to the sense of calm I felt on a date with someone else. For a whole week I told myself I was probably just "intimidated by them." I didn't realize it was a red flag, until someone told me a bad experience they had had with this person, and I said out loud, "Oh my god, *my body knew!*" Do I regret the date? Fuck NO! I gained wisdom!

We need to live and experience life to learn what certain feelings in our bodies mean. The wisdom we build from experience helps us to live the life we want to live. And if you don't have a fucking clue about what it is you want in life right now, I am unbelievably excited for you. Once you start to express yourself, ignore the voice of fear and dare to act against it, small clues will start to reveal themselves to you. Because now you are getting closer to your intuition, you will finally start to hear her whispers, guiding you where to go next.

THE WORLD WAS NOT DESIGNED FOR YOU, YOU NEED TO DESIGN YOUR OWN

It's time for us to retreat inward, to start inspecting our inner worlds, dismantle the limits we've created on what we're capable of, and design the lives we want from the inside *out* instead of reaching outside to fix the inside. Why? Because the "outside" was quite *literally* designed by men. Not just the systems, not just advertising, patriarchy, and capitalism, but even most of the streets, our religion, our democracy. In her book *Invisible Women*, Caroline Criado Perez unpacks the many ways women are forgotten entirely in the design of our world, where the "default" of our society is male, with drugs tested only on men, phones too big for women's hands, and cars designed for male bodies. Crash bags are tested exclusively on men, which is deadly for women since our legs are shorter, making us 17 percent more likely to die in

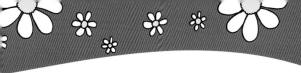

a car crash. In an interview about her book, Caroline said, "When you get an over-the-counter medication, it doesn't tell you male and female doses—it says 'child' and 'adult,' and that adult is a man. To me, that shows the scale of the problem we have here. All these drugs need to be looked at to see whether male and female doses should be different." We need new tools, and we're not going to find them outside us.

The world was mostly imagined by men. Men engineered capitalism, creating our daily habits as consumers through advertising, leaving us all wanting more and more and more, to the point where we are now destroying the earth and robbing her of resources to keep producing it all. The way the world looks is mostly a physical manifestation of the inner worlds of men. It is no exaggeration to say that our lives are the manifestation of the fiction of white men, from centuries ago, and the discomfort we feel in them is only multiplied when you introduce any further marginalization into a woman's life. The world was not built for us! We're living in what was once these men's dreams! The school systems, government, public transport, roads, none of this was considered with your needs in mind, because women were not designing them. The only public place designed for women is the fucking shopping mall! With "WOMEN" sections on the ground floor, the only time we are prioritized is when we are spending money on pretty things!

A big part of creating an expansive mindset is being an expansive *thinker*. We need to look beyond our current environment and act as audaciously as those whose dreams we are currently living in. It is a powerful experiment of curiosity to ask ourselves what our world would look like if we too believed we had the power to make it a physical manifestation of our own inner fictions. What if young girls were taught to allow themselves to dream as big as boys? I want you to know that your frustration at how everything somehow feels "too much" and "not enough" at the same time is a valid response from your body. Your body and mind are working in *exactly* the way our environment intends them to work—behaving as consumers who are never satisfied. You do not feel enough, because the world cannot handle people who do feel enough.

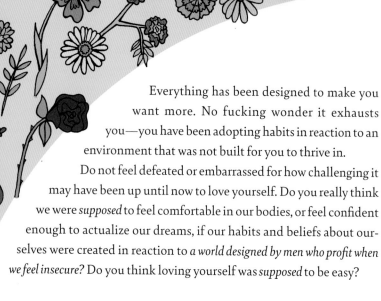

Everything has been designed to make you want more. No fucking wonder it exhausts you—you have been adopting habits in reaction to an environment that was not built for you to thrive in.

Do not feel defeated or embarrassed for how challenging it may have been up until now to love yourself. Do you really think we were *supposed* to feel comfortable in our bodies, or feel confident enough to actualize our dreams, if our habits and beliefs about ourselves were created in reaction to *a world designed by men who profit when we feel insecure?* Do you think loving yourself was *supposed* to be easy?

YOU ARE EXPANSIVE BY NATURE

This "shrinking" begins with the way we raise young girls. While boys are taught to get stuck in, get messy, and dream big, girls are often told that their appearance is the asset to strengthen. We encourage them to pour all of their attention, money, and the most finite, precious resource of time into how they look. Despite the best efforts of parents and teachers to encourage us to focus in school or pursue something beyond beauty, our actual day-to-day experience teaches us that people don't like bright girls, they like obedient girls. We are called annoying, stubborn, arrogant, bossy, and big-headed for daring to express ourselves, for trying, or being excellent at anything. And because we need to survive, we dim ourselves. We learn to play it small so we don't threaten the egos of the boys who we learn not to "outsmart." And though no one dares to say it out loud, we also learn that we must play it small so we don't threaten the other girls. Like a dimmable light bulb, we adjust our brightness accordingly so as not to outshine anyone else. This is a survival mechanism that, if not consciously shaken off, will follow us the rest of our lives.

We then grow into adult women who understand intuitively when to shrink and when to expand, internalizing the fear we learned as young girls of what others might do if we dare to surpass *their* limits. If you do not play it small in your industry, office, or family and you commit "the crime of outshining," your reputation is at risk.

For a lot of us, the mere threat of social rejection is too painful, and so we learn to stay small. We are raised to crave social acceptance, hooked on it like a drug since we're young girls with remarks, glares, and gestures we know are loaded with judgment and tell us how worthy or good we are. We learn quickly that prettiness and conformity is not a fun or playful form of self-expression, but a way to survive. We confine girls within the parameters of behavior we deem acceptable—submissive, pretty, thin, virginal, quiet, agreeable—training them by revoking praise the second they act out of line.

Known as relational aggression, this hits women where they hurt most—in their relationships. It is a form of social punishment and control we give girls for daring to shine "too bright." It looks like ignoring her on the playground when we normally play with her, not saving a seat in class, pretending she missed the invite to the sleepover. In adulthood, this looks like doing a group hang with the office girls on a night we know she's busy, cozying up with her enemy, spreading gossip about her under the disguise of "I'm just worried for her." All of this is designed to weaken the woman-who-dared-to-shine-too-bright's self-esteem, to get her to conform. This not only gets a woman to behave accordingly and mute her true self-expression, but she often believes it's all her fault and attempts to "make up for it" by trying harder, or grovelling and asking what she did wrong. Relational aggression preys on our social need to belong. We can clearly see how this works on social media: when we post something we love and believe in, but delete it because it doesn't get many likes and the ancient part of our brain fears being ostracized from the tribe because of our "unlikeability." Freedom is leaving that post up. Allowing our expression to stand its ground against fear of others not liking it. Life too has its own unpredictable algorithm where we cannot know how people will perceive us. We taste freedom when we realize fear has no control over how and when we show up. It is just fear. And we can ignore it.

When it comes to "why" we want women to shrink, I have often wondered if a lot of men's misogyny is fueled by an unconscious envy. A subconscious and repressed desire to be emotional, expressive, and vulnerable themselves. Because here's the thing: you don't feel the need to control something unless it's a threat. You don't need to control something unless the thing you are trying to cage is feared as being more powerful than you. We don't control weakness, we control *threats*. If femininity really was a weakness, it would not require such stealthy, repetitive, law-enforced taming to keep us submissive. If we were naturally so submissive, surely, our smallness would take care of itself? But it doesn't. Women *need* to be "controlled" and persuaded to be smaller versions of ourselves because our nature is to bloom, expand, and create—and that is a frightening reality to confront for people who like to keep those parts of themselves hidden.

A WOMAN IS NOT YOUR ENEMY, SHE IS YOUR INVITATION

Because of the closeness and intimacy we develop with other women, of course, the shrinking can and does take place here too. The programming we collectively receive to "be small" is a large part of why women can become so resentful of other women when they decide to bloom. *How dare she live outside the confines of womanhood?!* These women, confined in their own fear, often attempt to reclaim their diminished sense of power by *becoming* the cage for other women, shaming and judging them in the same way that society does to them. It is learned behavior. Their only association with power, is the power that has confined their own lives. To attain this power, they feel they must behave just like the men. If we're not conscious of it and our pain drives our lives around for us, we end up becoming the "cage" for other women. The "feel good" sensation we derive from putting another woman down becomes the crumbs we use to feed the insatiable void inside ourselves, to temporarily quiet its hunger. Until it wants something bigger...

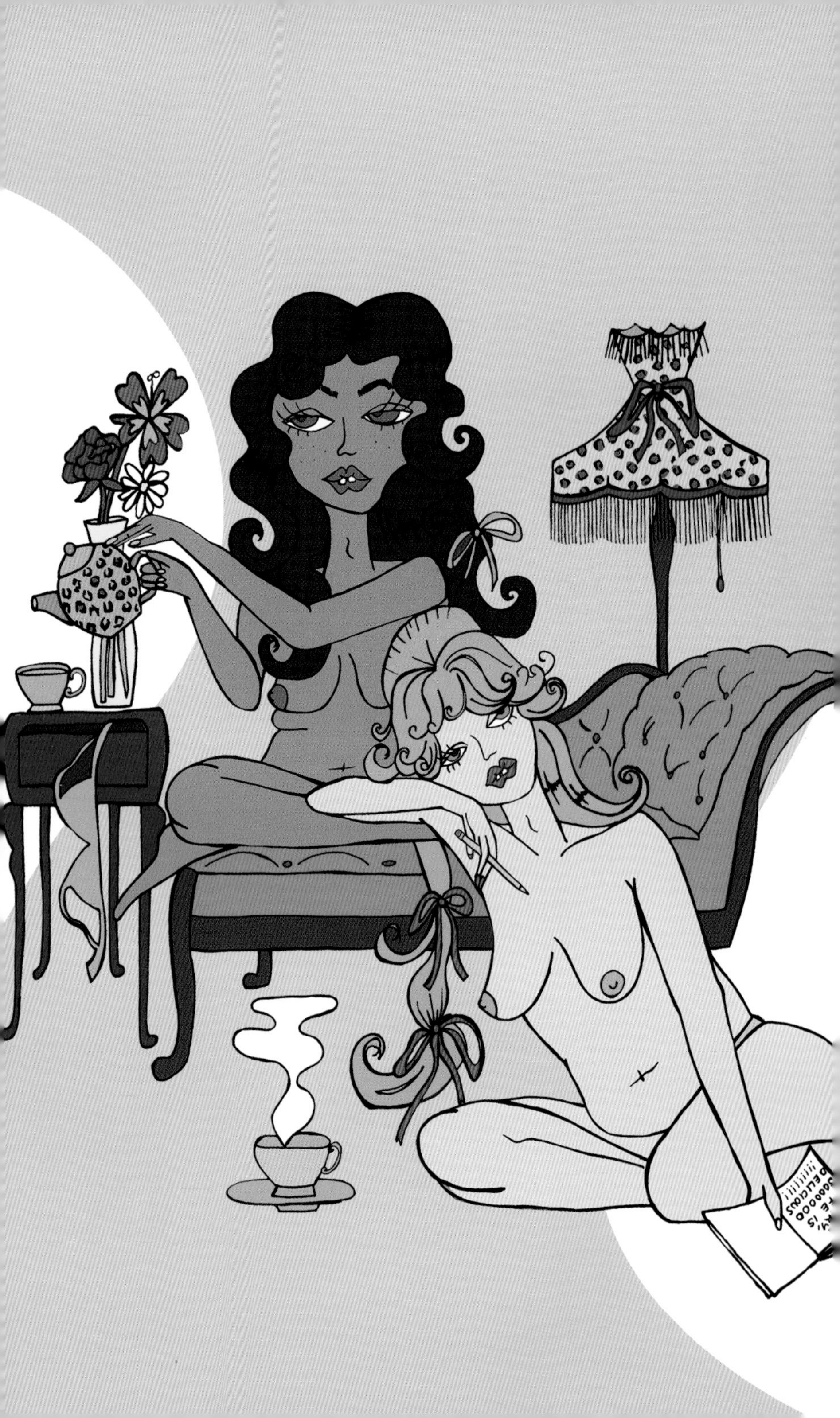

When we have been taught to make ourselves "small," seeing another woman living with reckless abandon, as though the limits that confine us in fear do not confine her, a woman with seemingly infinite amounts of joy, generosity, vitality, and happiness who acts *without* seeing the boundaries we live by, is going to trigger and hit that SMALL wound. *It's going to hurt us in that place we are aching to express, but we're taught to suppress.* And that stored expression we have repressed inside us, the resentment we have lodged inside ourselves, is going to come loose.

We might project our negative feelings onto her. *How unfair! How dare she? She's so annoying, why does she get to be so free and expressive? She makes me feel so SHIT. Who does she think she is?* What we do with that triggered pain when we feel it is **crucial**. We can either choose to view her freedom as an invitation and to step out of our cage, or repeat what has been done to us—shame her in the hopes that we can put her light out and get her to join us in misery, behind the limits that confine us. Most of us don't see this choice because—and I cannot emphasize this enough—until we are conscious of something and can hold it up to the light, we cannot change it. It lurks in the control room of our minds, in our deep subconscious, pulling the levers of our behavior. It is only by shining a light on it that we can notice when it is taking over and possessing us, that we can realize what's happening and put ourselves in charge of it.

That woman who triggers us is only serving as a mirror to our own fear. But when we do not like what we see, when we see the gap between who we *want* to be and who we *are*, instead of looking inward at ourselves, we may focus our pain unfairly on her. We might even recruit others to join us shaming her, in order to numb our feelings of discomfort. We do this without realizing that all we are defending is the limitation of our own self-expression. We hold on to our cage when we do this. In setting limits for others and how they are able to express themselves, shaming women under the guise of wanting what's "best for her" or what's "best for feminism," we reinforce those limits for ourselves too and hold on to our pain. *A cage on you is a cage on me. But at least we're both caged together,* our wounded, SMALL selves tell us. This is known as "crabs in a

bucket" syndrome. Crabs, when they are
caught at sea, have a chance of survival by helping one another escape out of the bucket. But the second
one crab tries to escape and gets close, the crabs work together
to bring it down, ending in their collective demise—*if I can't escape, neither can you!* But here's where it gets interesting: crabs don't
naturally live in buckets. When we see them in their natural habitat, they
are collaborative. It's the unknown, frightening, and limiting environment
of the bucket that makes them behave against their instincts, turning against
one another in this unfamiliar environment. The same is true for humans.
Capitalism, patriarchy, and every system of oppression is our "bucket," forcing us all to abandon our collaborative nature for one of competitiveness for
survival. But we are a naturally collaborative species, it's how we have come so
far! We do not need to compete and, just like the crabs, become territorial and
fearful and tear each other down. We have forgotten an essential truth—that
if the crabs worked together, they could collectively escape.

When we witness a woman trying to escape that bucket, succeed, go beyond her SMALL limits, we have a choice between joining her and facing the
same criticism and shame, staying quiet, or dragging her down and remaining
caged. None of these options sound good, *but only one of them leads to freedom.*
In bringing other women back down with us—through gossip, shaming,
exclusion—we cling onto our pain too, we stay in the bucket. It puts a temporary plaster on our own pain. We get to avoid the reflection. We feel a weird
sense of belonging in joining in with others in common, sadistic cause. But we
must look for a different option. We must look for the only option that leads
to freedom, by feeling the pain ourselves rather than inflicting it on others.
We must choose to view it as an opportunity to release our SMALL training,
an opportunity to leap into expansion. To shed our limits!

We can't rely on other women also having this collaborative mindset before we do it ourselves. We may find that we are burned many times by women
who do not wish us to succeed or be happy the same way, even when we help
them, even when we support them—and it hurts. It's shit. There's no other

way to put it. But that does not mean we stop fucking growing, on our own, with or without them, or that we stop trying to climb out of that bucket. The irony is, other women will still benefit. Because our freedom from shame and fear contributes on a scale felt by everyone. Even if they do not want to join us, by continuing to evolve and heal and better our lives, we contribute to women's freedom as a whole.

The first way we can begin to challenge these sadistic urges is to question the voice in our heads. What is it inside us that wants to lunge out and drag her back behind that line with us, standing next to us in the cage of fear? Whose voice is that? Is it the same voice that punished us when we tried to express ourselves?

Stop being so loud.

Stop doing that, it's embarrassing.

You're too much, that's so cringe.

She's so annoying, why does she get to be everything she wants?

Must be nice for some!

When we feel an urge to lunge out and judge, we have detected something within us that we were taught to be ashamed of. Rather than perceiving her as a threat, we can see her as a fucking invitation. If we pause and observe that she is not hurting us, that it's an old story and old pain that is hurting, she becomes our freedom, our permission slip to step courageously over that line we have been taught not to cross and join her in being authentically ourselves. When you witness a woman living courageously, try to see it as permission for you to expand beyond your own limits TOO.

WE'RE *JUST* LIKE THE OTHER GIRLS

I've noticed something sneaky happening with women's envy and jealousy towards one another. Just as patriarchy has evolved its tactics to control women to be less obvious, the ways that *women* seek to control other women have evolved, and it's just as insidious. It is no longer considered politically correct for us to comment on another woman's appearance. We will be ac-

cused by others of not being a
"girls' girl"—we will be accused of
being anti-feminist. While this is great
and creates an awareness of how we discuss
other women, it does not address the root issue of
why we feel the need to do this to them and, rather, it only serves to shame
the "form" our judgment takes! So, although degrading slurs based on a
woman's appearance are becoming less common (in public at least), that
doesn't mean the reactive and ugly urge to judge other women has disap-
peared, or that doing it has stopped. It has merely evolved and changed its
face, delivering the same poison designed to weaken their image, just harder
to detect. Judging and slagging off women hasn't gone anywhere, we have
merely shifted from a woman's appearance to her morals. It just became
political!

We have discovered a new, more acceptable, and "feminist" way to shame
women publicly now without facing any consequences, because we wrap it up
inside moral righteousness. We've just started calling each other "problematic" instead. This is just another way to shame a woman for her lack of moral
purity, smearing her character in an instant with a word no one ever wants
to be associated with. The word claws and hooks into our good-girl training
and makes us feel like the devil. It is the modern-day equivalent of "witch."
Branding a woman with this vague label is the perfect trap because if you
decide to defend her, or even ask, "What did she actually do wrong?"—you
too may be considered problematic for even asking. You too may face social
exclusion. You're expected to just go along with it.

Of course, judging women's appearance is still rampant. It is still alive
and thriving. But where we cannot get away with this, we may give it a morally righteous makeover and find we are even "praised" for putting another
woman down because it appears to be out of our "concern" for her. If we
never address the root cause of why we want to judge other women and heal
it, the judging will never stop. It will always evolve to become more and
more undetected, because it is still fulfilling a need inside us—the need to

feel bigger, better, more than someone. It is ugly but important work that is never finished.

I say this as someone who deeply believes in accountability, in pulling each other aside to say, "Babe, I love you, and I think this can be handled better." But I do not believe in shaming , or policing each other into becoming impossibly perfect and saying all the right things all the time. We will never be able to live this way. I do not say all the right things, and I don't fucking want to! I want to be human.

I've also participated in the gossiping about other women, discussing my "concern" for them and immediately feeling a stinky, thick, potent shame for doing it. The truth is, any time I have done this was because I had not yet come to terms with my own imperfections, and this unaddressed shame manifested as an outward attack on the woman who reminded me of my own private, personal flaws. In shaming her, I was trying to avoid the shame I felt in myself. The shame of simply being imperfect.

If we genuinely want people to be better, shaming is not the answer. Fear is not a sustainable fuel for growth—love is. And if we can learn, slowly, to love ourselves with all our limits and our moral imperfections, we find that it is easier to love other women. EVEN the morally imperfect ones who don't get everything right all the time. Just like you. Just like all of us. You *are* just like the other girls. We all are.

The internet has become a particularly ugly place for our negativity to dwell and thrive because it has the potential for enormous and instant rewards. The instant gratification of expressing negativity and having it receive attention, filling us with the digital warmth of social validation, is slowly robbing us of the chance to use our uncomfortable emotions to reflect on ourselves and our inner worlds. The gratification we receive when we gossip about someone online or to our friends and gorge on juicy details is more instant than if we shut up and consider the root of why this person brings out such a strong reaction in us. I can't count the number of times I have reached for my phone in the past when I should have just reached for my diary. Just because we think something and a bunch of other insecure people agree with us, that does not mean it's rooted in any truth. We want so badly to escape the discomfort of sitting with our pain that it's all too easy to just reach for the quick solution.

But when we choose to wait before responding to our envy, or any emotion, we can start to see the shape the issue is taking not outside us, but within us. To paraphrase Carl Jung's teachings, "What you resist, persists." By continuing to see our demons as outside us and not something to be exorcized from within, soon another demon will pop up, presenting us with the same deep-seated inadequacies we felt before. If we keep pointing outside, we avoid the truth inside.

But guess what? It's not always internalized misogyny. Any time I talk about internalized misogyny and how, sometimes, we might not like a woman because she reminds us of what we wish we could be, I say it with fear that the people-pleaser, the doormat, the chronically self-reflective woman, may use this to further erase and ignore the intuition she feels about a woman who is actually being mean to her, something her gut has accurately picked up on. Being able to discern whether the way we feel about a woman is about "our stuff" or "her stuff," whether our gut is accurately picking up on strange

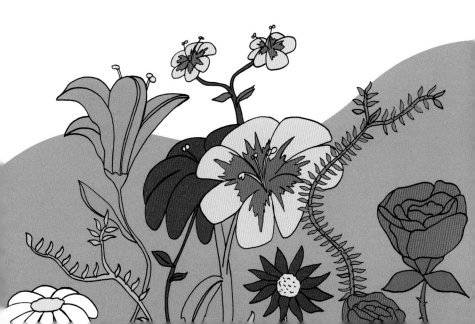

glances, on odd behavior from her, is not always clear. We will delve deeper into how to connect to our intuition later. But generally, if we feel unnecessarily defensive, overly critical, or are making snap and harsh judgments about a person, it is likely a projection of OUR stuff. It almost sounds like a little child inside us—*That's not fair! Why her? She's so annoying! Why does she get to do these things?* For me, intuition tends to be a quieter nagging.

I fucking love women. My love for women is the guiding force for everything I do. Women are my fucking muse, and I want to slowly contribute to a world in which we no longer feel we are fighting for space, but "lifting as we climb." Because that is our fucking nature. Look at what happens when women hang out in their own private spaces, in their bedrooms, or share private moments in the absence of men, in the absence of status, in the absence of competition. We are collaborative. So we can give each other a look when our ex enters the party, or a quick glance when we want to leave. We watch each other's drinks with the vigilance of a hired private security guard, we compliment girls on their makeup and watch in awe as our moms, sisters, partners, and friends get ready in their bedrooms. These are the moments when the façade comes down. This is our nature. *This is how the crabs behave when they're out of the bucket.* I do not mean to paint a romanticized image of women without men as "perfect." As a queer woman I can tell you it's far from the truth, and there can be just as much competition in a lesbian bar. But when we have our own private moments together, we feel less restriction on our true selves. With courage, we can start to bring our true selves outside, and slowly, the world will no longer feel like a bucket in which we are forced to compete. In which we are forced to be small and pull others down.

Breaching the limits that have confined us within the parameters of smallness, that have taught us to shrink ourselves for safety, feels deeply uncomfortable. You are about to EXPAND and stretch beyond them. Growing pains are to be expected. Even if you desire to reach your potential and feel very fucking serious about doing this, the voice in your mind is still going to be screaming at you every step of the way, telling you to come back behind those lines, that the world is a frightening place and that you will never be able to handle it. It's not going anywhere just because you want it to.

What better way to control an entire population of people than to convince them to cringe and fear the part of themselves that will set them free? Femininity and intuition are powerful beyond measure. It is why we are all taught to fear and control them.

In the next chapter, I'm going to warn you about a little trap you might stumble upon when you wake up to the ways you have been "shrinking" yourself. As debilitating as it is to shrink, there *is* such a thing as too much expansion. Let's look at the seductive trap of hyper-independence, and how I fell for it myself.

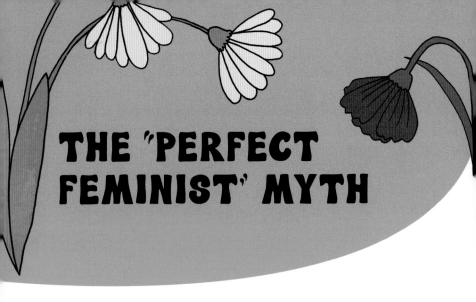

THE 'PERFECT FEMINIST' MYTH

There's a little patriarchal trap I hadn't noticed until I fell right into it. It's hiding within the feminist movement, masking itself as "liberation"—like a wolf in sheep's clothing. You might have fallen for it yourself—the seductive trap of becoming hyper-independent.

When I left a toxic relationship, I unshackled myself from a small and fearful life and unleashed the repressed feminist rage in me that ached to lunge out. It was the rage I never felt safe to express in moments when my body was violated and my limits crossed, the moments I did not feel safe enough to assert myself, when my ideas were belittled and I did not defend them. The times I lied to protect the reputation of someone who was hurting me. Years of pent-up self-expression poured out into this gushing, chaotic, beautiful, feminist anger. I vowed to become as independent as possible and galvanize other women to stand up for themselves too. The title of the diary I started at the time was literally *PERPETUALLY EXHAUSTED BY MEN*. I hated them. And I loved it. Hating men in my head and my diary was the closest thing I could feel to having power over them, in a life where I had frustratingly experienced having very little. What I didn't prepare for was that hating men would become just as exhausting as my years of mentally submitting to them.

By rebelling against the men who had hurt me and the patriarchal structures that have held women back for centuries—with a *fuck everyone, fuck this, fuck that, I don't need help* attitude—I didn't realize, until it was too late and I burned out, that I had started to replicate the same hyper-independent cage that ensnares men to their toxic masculinity. The patriarchal trap that prevents *men* from being able to express themselves, ask for help, cry, and indulge in and express their emotions. On my trajectory towards becoming an independent woman who relied on no one, I accidentally ended up denying the sensitive, feminine, and playful half of myself, the same way that men are encouraged to. Vulnerability became a sign of weakness, I became defensive at the suggestion that I might need to rest, someone offering me "help" made me feel insulted that they thought I couldn't do it on my own, I lost myself in work and productivity and neglected my body's screams to slow down. Patriarchy discredited vulnerability and slowly I discredited it within myself, albeit in the name of becoming an "independent woman." If we're not careful, this desire to unshackle ourselves from an oppressive structure to prove that we can do it all on our own can end up coming full circle, going so far that it becomes oppressive again.

In the words of Carl Jung, "You always become the thing you fight the most." Despite my intentional rebellion against patriarchy, I had started to embody it. *How the fuck did that happen?!*

Hyper-independence became a form of self-protection. My brain decided "fuck this!" and closed up the walls of my heart to protect me. What made it trickier to notice was that "independence" is something we praise women for as a progressive quality, particularly within feminism. A trauma response very common in people who have been betrayed or hurt in their relationships is to become the direct opposite of who they were when they were hurt. But the truth is, we do not shame these feminine parts of ourselves because they are "weak," but because they are vulnerable and at times frightening to embody. We shame the parts of ourselves that are silly, feminine, vulnerable, and open—because it is likely that we were hurt when we expressed these things. These parts can then start to feel unsafe to show. When you have been hurt by someone, or by multiple people, when you rightfully mourn the years of your girlhood and womanhood that were lost to fear, pain, and hurt, the inner bodyguard steps in, protecting your softness, refusing anyone access to it, and vowing to never be hurt again. This is necessary for a period, but if we don't remove that bodyguard when we no longer need it, we can remain in a state of defense for months or even years without realizing it. We become hardened. It becomes who we are. Our life becomes a resistance to vulnerability. We live in survival mode. We avoid our softness. Our femininity. Our openness. Our playful carefree selves. We stop engaging with the world. The hopeful part of us that once saw beauty in life becomes replaced with cynicism, seriousness, hyper-vigilance, and caution. We create an entire personality built around defending those vulnerable parts from being exposed. Just like men have done, protecting the façade they're taught to craft, of their "masculinity." Without our awareness, our brains learn that to be safe in this world means to avoid being that open person again. Our brains fear it was the "back door" we left open in our lives that allowed someone in. So they close it. Board it up. Building hard walls around ourselves to protect us instead.

But this rejection of our softness becomes its own cage. I had seen men live like this, and I didn't want to live like that myself. I had seen how repressive and exhausting the pressure of being hyper-independent can be. It was lonely. I didn't want to close myself off from the realm of feeling, delighting, the realm of connection where life happens. I had to learn to integrate the parts of myself that were buried beneath shame. To examine the ways in which I had shamed vulnerability within myself. The desire to do everything by ourselves and become too independent strips us of the beautiful warmth and connection built in asking others for help, it stops us living, building communities, it robs us of the wonderful realm of feeling, delighting, and enjoying, laughing, dancing, singing, crying. By shutting ourselves off after trauma, we no longer expose ourselves to joy. If we leave the walls up for too long, we

forget that they need to come
down for anything beautiful to visit us. To
be touched and delighted by life in the ways we will
discuss in this book, we need to remain open.

WHY IS HYPER-INDEPENDENCE SO SEDUCTIVE?

The idea of being independent is not toxic. Historically—and still in many places today—women have had to ask their husbands or their fathers for permission to do just about anything. In fact, it wasn't long ago that women were still considered to be the actual property of men, and passages in the Old Testament state that if a man rapes an unmarried virgin, then he must pay money to *her father* as compensation for having ruined his "property." Women have "belonged" to men for centuries. Lived in their shadows. Existed as their property like cattle. Relied on them for access to money and power, food, shelter, and survival. Many women still rely on men today, some in horrendously abusive relationships, for access to power. Until 1974, a woman in the US still wasn't able to apply for a credit card without a male guarantor! If we look across the span of human history, women have been made to rely on men for thousands of years. Today, women are only at the very beginning of tasting a smidgen of freedom from men and considering what might be possible. We do not yet know just how delicious it can get.

It is no surprise then that the counterculture that formed in response to thousands of years of being oppressed, controlled, and dominated was to swing the pendulum in the other direction and to try to be as "free" as fucking possible. Except, the only role models most of us had for "freedom" and success were men. A lot of us had to imitate them to be taken seriously in the man's world of work. But the trouble is, men don't have everything figured out, either. Quite the opposite. Men are socialized to suppress vulnerability and emulate the façade that they have it all together—*and that is what kills them.* That is why they kill each other. That is why, according to a UN report, 96 percent of all violent crime is committed by men. In spite of the freedom and privileges men collectively have, their way of being in the world is far from something to admire, let alone something we should be encouraged to imitate. The only model we previously had to look up to for freedom and independence was toxic as fuck.

In women, the glamorization of constant hustle, coupled with the ruthless ambition we feel we need to emulate in a "man's world," has been named "Girl Boss feminism." But it's deeper than being a "Girl Boss." I know from experience that most people who refuse to rest and refuse to slow down at the expense of their health are normally outrunning something. Someone who refuses to stop, literally feels like they can't. It's such a fucking effective and even seductive way of escaping vulnerability. If we never slow down, we never have to feel hurt. If we keep working, we will receive more rewards and validation to temporarily fill the void. If we say we don't have "time" for real relationships, we never have to be vulnerable enough for someone to hurt us again. But what if we don't have to hustle all the time? What if we can slow down?

HOW HAS TOXIC MASCULINITY MANIFESTED WITHIN YOU?

So much of feminism is focused on taking stock of the ways we are harmed by men, that we can often glaze over the ways we have adopted parts of toxic masculinity ourselves. In a world that demands invulnerability and toughness from everyone to survive, it is inevitable it will leave traces within us. Trying to be perfect by chasing, striving to prove our worth, and hustling to receive approval and love isn't liberation. It is just patriarchy in a pair of heels and a pantsuit, trying to seduce us to become just as closed off and afraid of vulnerability as men. Perfection is a myth. It does not exist. The perfect woman, the perfect feminist, none of it is real. We exhaust ourselves until we can no longer move trying to achieve it. There is a cost for trying to be perfect at anything. It requires a complete obliteration of our limits. Sleep. Happiness. Quality time with people we love. Our health. My body has taught me that my limits are not an "obstacle" to overcome, but that these limits are my body's wisdom.

I've been asked by people, "What do you think about feminists who take

STRIVING, PROVING AND **HUSTLING** TO RECEIVE **APPROVAL** ISN'T **LIBERATION**, IT IS JUST **PATRIARCHY** IN A **PAIR** OF **HEELS** AND A **PANT SUIT.**

it too far?" Honestly, I think every feminist has the right to take it "too far." Don't you want to take it "too far" after reading that 96 percent statistic above? Every new and unfurling feminist has the right to be messy in her revelations for a little while. We need to have the room to work it all out, to fumble around with this new freedom, to express and to grieve for the years we lost to fear and the frustration that as long as there are men on the streets we will always be walking around with a degree of hyper-vigilance for the rest of our lives. The grief of realizing we were measuring our worth against a set of beauty ideals that change every day and were created to the detriment of our happiness and invented to slow us down. When we wake up to this for the first time, a beautiful, righteous anger is born. I was a proper little shit after my feminist awakening, starting debates over breakfast and snapping at people if there was even a whiff of misogyny. Although it was gut-wrenchingly painful to realize the world was not as I thought, I am grateful the feminist movement provided the perfect refuge for me to express my rage productively, turning it into action, galvanizing others and creating real change. We all deserve the room to express this. We all deserve to expel the pain from our bodies and our lives, the pain we had learned to suppress.

The trouble is, if we stay in this state for too long, we burn out. Rage is a great catalyst, but it is not a sustainable fuel. In the words of Glennon Doyle, "*Rebellion is as much of a cage as obedience is.* They both mean living in reaction to someone else's way instead of forging your own." Rebelling against the things that hurt us—whether it's patriarchy, our parents, an ex, an old bully—becomes another cage. Because our new identity is forged out of a constant opposition to something, our new identity relies on our pain to exist. By running *from* something, in trying to prove *someone* wrong, in trying to earn the love *from* someone we never received through chasing accomplishments, we still remain attached to it. We never actually get to heal as long as part of us still yearns for the people that hurt us to see how much pain they caused. If part of us still relies on an apology from them to move on. In my constant "attack" mode of calling things out, pointing the finger at men, closing myself off to love, the rage and pain I felt from people who had hurt me was still woven into my identity, and it was impossible to move beyond it. It stopped me from enjoying my life.

The only way I could move on from my pain was to release the identity I had created in opposition and resistance to it. To denounce neither "feminism" nor "patriarchy" but to take everything back to basics and start from scratch asking, "Who am I without my pain?" To bring that pendulum back to the middle point and find my own fucking voice. It took burning out to be able to finally see that there was nothing wrong with my softness, that my femininity wasn't the problem, my ability to see the best in people wasn't the problem, that there was nothing embarrassing about expressing myself. I realized that, far more brave than suppressing these qualities, was the courageous choice to dare to love and be open to experiencing life again, even after the trauma. That there is actually nothing more courageous than *remaining* a soft and open woman, in spite of what has happened to you. To do the work it takes to let go, to transcend the pain and REFUSE to allow it to harden you the way it has hardened men. To become a free woman in her power, *without* exhausting herself. To remain soft, open, loving, passionate, vulnerable, and trust that you will be fine if it doesn't turn out the way you hoped. To not define the parts of you that allow you to feel EVERYTHING as "weak." It turns out I didn't need to abandon my softness or build walls around her, what I needed was actively to build trust with my OWN opinion of who was a person worthy of gaining access to her. I just needed to learn to listen to my own intuition and to stop outsourcing my decisions to others. It was the only way I would learn how to discern people's characters.

DO NOT MAKE OTHER PEOPLE YOUR COMPASS

The temptation to outsource our power by allowing others to decide what's best for us and silence our intuition is everywhere. When we're looking for answers or trying to discover our purpose in life, many of us turn towards feminism, religion, podcasts, therapists, or figures of authority. You might have even picked up this book for that reason! To engage with other people's voices in a healthy way is to allow them to guide us back to discovering our own intuition. The trap I and many others have fallen into is using other people to replace it.

That is exactly what I did when I stopped trying to model the "perfect woman" and began trying to model the "perfect feminist." I had once again handed over the keys of my life to an external voice and allowed it to tell me who to be. I had given the power of my self-perception and my values over to something else. To avoid the trap of giving someone or something the power to dictate our inner voice, we need to learn the sound of our own.

I had outsourced my intuition and allowed other people to tell me what was right and wrong, even what was right and wrong about myself, for many years. So obsessed with being morally perfect to the point it would haunt me, I found myself apologizing for things I didn't do and censoring myself to be the most palatable and least offensive version possible. I was a shell of the woman I knew I could be, because I didn't have the courage to trust that my own opinion of myself was worth anything. Years of abusive relationships had swamped my ability to test what was real and what was false. When we don't trust ourselves and begin searching for answers, we are particularly vulnerable to being swept up into other people's persuasive ideology. Whether that's a friend, a cult, a religion, a political party, or even the charm of a stranger on a date. "If you stand for nothing, you'll fall for anything," the saying goes. Even if it's not harmful, even if the ideology is "good," if you're not careful you may find yourself leaving one toxic environment only to seek refuge in a space where you live by another set of strict rules. This has nothing to do with intelligence. It is often the simple and earnest mistake of believing that everyone tells the truth about who they are, and that other people have answers you cannot find within yourself.

In her essay "*Trashing: The Dark Side of Sisterhood*" Jo Freeman says of feminism: "The Movement seduced me by its sweet promise of sisterhood. It claimed to provide a haven from the ravages of a sexist society; a place where one would be understood. It was my very need for feminism that made me vulnerable. I gave the movement the right to

STOP TRYING TO WIN AT OTHER PEOPLE'S GAMES AND CREATE YOUR OWN!

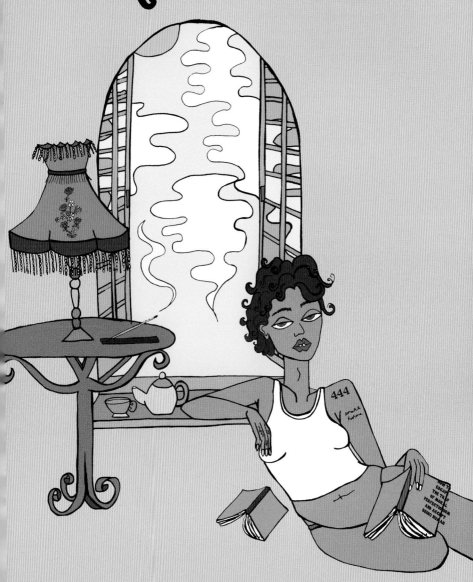

judge me because I trusted it. And when it judged me worthless, I accepted that judgment."

The moment we hand over our self-worth and judgment to someone else, we give them the most unbelievable amount of power. We make them into our punishing god—someone who can scold us or praise us based on "good" or "bad" behavior. They can give us happiness, or they can take it away by telling us that we did something wrong. This training shapes our behavior, just as we have discussed patriarchy has done to women.

Moral perfectionism and purity plagues women's minds, perhaps as deeply if not more deeply than our need to be pretty. Moral perfection has always been expected of women, but its modern conception has become stealthier. As we discussed, the old and outdated way of shaming women to remain small by attacking them superficially for their appearance is being replaced with a new method: we can now scare women into being small and quiet by making them terrified of saying the wrong thing and being judged as morally evil because of it. There was a time when women were not allowed to have opinions, now we must have the correct ones. This is how patriarchy has seeped its way into feminism. It doesn't even need to get its hands dirty from silencing us anymore. It sits back relaxing in a chair with its legs spread wide, whisky in hand, watching us for sport, as we scold and punish each other, scaring one another into the smallest possible versions of ourselves. This new, impossible moral standard for us to live up to is just another way to grind us down, keep us small, and exhaust us. How can we possibly focus on expressing ourselves authentically if our output is being filtered through the lens of whether or not it will be correct enough? Good enough? Moral enough? It is the reason many people decide it's simply not worth the hassle and decide to stop sharing their thoughts.

BECOME YOUR OWN FUCKING COMPASS

We need to be careful that a desire for community or a sense of belonging, even within a movement as progressive as feminism, does not have us accidentally replicating the same cage we just broke free from. Just because something sounds great, sounds "right," we still need to learn to think for ourselves. When I was trying to heal, trying to figure out who I was as a woman in the world, outside of who it had told me to be, I found a community in feminism. It spoke to my soul, and it still does. It disrupted everything I had been taught a woman needed to be—small. There was space for me within feminism to finally be big, loud, confident. But, as I slowly learned through random forms of punishment, not *too* confident. Not *too* big. Not *too* intelligent. The ways I was being made to become smaller within feminism started to sound very familiar to the ways I had been made to feel small by men and the media. Like Jo Freeman, slowly the desire for community, acceptance, and purpose I sought in feminism meant that I made it my new moral compass. It could tell me if I was worthy or unworthy. It could tell me to "*be quiet and listen*" or "*speak out, right now!*" and I was ready, like a good girl, waiting for the orders. Though the face of the entity that was now controlling my life had changed no longer a man, no longer patriarchy—I was still looking for answers everywhere but in myself. I didn't know how to think for myself. I had found another value system which I felt I had to live by, once again giving away my personal power to something else telling me to be SMALL.

YOU ARE THE DIRECTOR OF YOUR LIFE

- *Don't do that, it's embarrassing.*
- *Do you think anyone will care about your work?*
- *Remember the last time you tried to dance? EMBARRASSING.*
- *Look how amazing she looks. You will never look that good.*
- *Don't cancel tonight, they won't invite you to anything else. Suck it up and go.*
- *You don't deserve to find love.*
- *You are disgusting, why bother leaving the house?*
- *Nothing good will ever happen to you.*

Most of us have a voice in our head, a running commentary, an inner monologue. It tells us what to do, what not to do, what to think about others. On occasion it will bring up random things from the past and drag us down, or predict things happening in the future to cause us great anxiety. This voice can either expand us and encourage us to go for the things we want to in life, or shrink us, hold us back, bully us, and make us stay SMALL.

In the words of Michael Singer, "There is nothing more important to true growth than realizing you are not the voice of the mind—you are the one who hears it." True freedom lies in knowing that whatever this voice says, it doesn't fucking matter. Because the voice is not *you*. You are not the repulsive thoughts you have, but the one who is *repulsed*. You are not the thoughts making judgments about others, you are the one watching them happen. You do not have to be held captive by the voice, because it is not who you are. It's like a scared, easily startled, out-of-control person.

Look inside yourself now, pause. Is it saying anything right now? Can you locate it? Is it saying, *"What is she on about?"* What startles the voice to start talking negatively? Does it happen under stress? When you make a mistake, does the voice punish you? Does it sound like a particular person you know?

I noticed that this voice tends to creep into my head precisely when I'm about to do something that will expand me. Going for dinner alone. Posting something online. Asking someone to be my friend. Walking into a fancy restaurant. Getting up to dance. Contributing to a group conversation. This critical voice lingers at the edge of my limits, at the edge of comfort, at the edge of familiarity. Threatening to strike me and keep me in line. To keep me small. *Don't say that, everyone will laugh at you! Stay home, it's better here! Don't go to a gig on your own, that's embarrassing.* For far too long, I lived my life obeying that voice because what I didn't know is that this voice is not making *demands*, it is making suggestions. Suggestions I could decline. I had the choice to say, "No," this whole time.

The next time the voice starts piping up in your head, can you make an effort to simply notice it, perhaps even give it a name to belittle it and remove its power? Snooty bum bum? *Grumpy Gail*? This will help you realize it is not in fact "you." It becomes a lot easier to ignore, and even laugh at, if you can imagine it as a different person, something separate to yourself. Which it is!

True freedom lies in knowing that this voice is not *you*. It sounds like you and it even uses your voice. But it isn't you. It's a broken record. When we're obsessed with something, we often say, "Oh my god, [insert book, sentence, outfit, film, TV series] is living rent free in my head!" But it's not just our individual obsessions that "live rent free" in our minds—the voice itself, the one that is *obsessing* over the obsessions, is living rent free. It's Grumpy Gail! Saboteur Sally! Downer Debs! The narrator. The commentator. The critic. The good news is, every time you ignore it, wear the thing you want, share your work, approach someone you're attracted to, ask someone to be your friend, set boundaries—you take a step towards freedom from that voice controlling you. You can starve it of attention, just as you would treat a bully.

You can prove that the voice is actually a coward, that it has no power over your life. You can learn to laugh at it when it gets grumpy, really, laugh at it! Piss it off with your indifference to it. Let it squirm in frustration as it watches how unbothered you are by it. No one gets to tell you when your life is over. Not the voice in your head. Not the fear caused by your trauma. Not your pain. Not the inner council of voices hell-bent on keeping you small, piping up to protect you from being hurt. The only person that can keep you small is you. You are the judge of this council. You get the final say.

TRANSCENDING FEAR IS THE BEST HIGH ON EARTH

I was a teenager when I realized that the voice in my head was a coward and that I *could* challenge it. The experience of challenging it was so profoundly blissful that I have only in recent years found the language to explain it, but I believe this moment changed my life forever. It was my first step out of living a life of fear. At fifteen, I had become so fed up that I found myself in the self-development section of a bookstore: I was experiencing a lot of anxiety and fear about what others thought of me, I had shortness of breath, heart palpitations, and felt harassed by the constant stream of panic in my mind. I found a book on mindfulness which encouraged the idea of *deliberately* stepping out of your comfort zone—an idea that rattled the anxious controlling perfectionist in me to the core. I felt like the book was calling me to step into a ring of fire.

One afternoon I went for a walk and passed a lush green field drenched in sunlight in the middle of a park. Every single cell in my body urged me to go and lie in the middle of this sunny, delicious patch of grass. But then I saw dog walkers. Girls the same age as me. Other teenagers. That fearful voice in my head piped up, telling me that it was embarrassing, that it was cringey. *Those dog walkers over there are going to laugh at you. What if the girls from your school find you and torment you?* The knots in my stomach clenched, my heart pounded, and I felt deeply uncomfortable, as if I was in actual danger. But I remembered my intention for going on the walk, and the wisdom of my book emerged as a new voice to challenge it: *stepping out of your comfort zone is the path to growth and freedom*. And so, disobeying the screams of the fearful voice, I thought I would try something new—doing something that scared me. I walked over to the middle of that field, lay back in the sunlight with my headphones on, and stared in awe at the sky. In that moment I felt like I was capable of anything. I had tasted what it was like to live a life beyond fear! Suddenly I realized I was not held captive by the voice in my head. I discovered that my life belonged to me. *That the voice of fear is a fucking suggestion, not a demand.*

After that, I knew that I was more powerful than this inner voice, because something inside me had overpowered it, something joyful that yearned to live *beyond* fear, to live deliciously and bask in that fucking sun on my own.

Since then, I have lost and rediscovered this connection to my joy. After experiencing trauma in my life, I stopped having as much courage to challenge the critical voices in my head and I began to believe them again. This inner council became more and more convincing, I allowed them to make the final call. I watched as the girl who had discovered a potent lust for life became a woman who could no longer get out of bed. Where I once saw possibilities for growth, I had started to see opportunities for failure. I lost my confidence. My morning routine consisted of screaming into my pillows at the weight of the responsibilities I didn't have the energy for and the self-care I could not muster the energy to do. I stopped reaching out, I stopped turning towards life. I stopped expressing myself. I stopped daring to step outside my comfort zone. Stopped dancing. Stopped listening to music. Stopped going on walks. Stopped laughing. Stopped being the person I once was. I watched as my life slowly took on the default shape of my fears, instead of being carved out intentionally by my desires and the things that brought me alive.

Every time I listened to the inner critic and endorsed those thoughts with my behavior by shrinking, dieting, punishing myself, perfecting, staying home, not expressing boundaries, and "going with the flow," I gave the negative voice in my mind more and more power. One by one, these choices diluted the potency of my life and left in their wake a watered-down, unrecognizable version of myself. I became the total sum product of everything I was afraid of and everything other people wanted me to be, instead of the architect of a life full of everything that I loved. Even after years of healing, leaving toxic relationships, it appeared that the last captor I had to defeat was the one within myself. After a full physical burnout, my body finally screamed at me: *You can't keep going on like this.*

BARRIERS TO BEING THE DIRECTOR

Being present is accessible to everyone, but our ability to acknowledge this inner voice in the first place can be blocked by the stress of our *outside* world, making it more challenging for some than others, depending on your responsibilities, your identity, your financial situation, and whether or not the relationships you're in are safe. For those who face poverty, racism, sexism, subjugation, and systems of oppression, this work may pose a tougher challenge. But these injustices can also act as a catalyst to change.

All of our time is tied up differently. The more responsibilities we have, the more stress we're likely to feel! The less access we have to our inner space, the further away we are pulled from the ability to consider "how" we are living. But what I hope to show you through this book is that being present isn't about needing to "do" more. It's shifting *how* we do it. One step at a time. It can be as accessible as simply taking a breath and using that moment to remind ourselves that we are not this voice of fear.

The journey back to mental freedom lies in reminding ourselves that no matter what the voice tells us, we must step out into the sun, seek out our small pleasures, dance again, say "no," take a deep breath when that fearful voice kicks in, to bring us back into reality, relax our nervous systems, and tell our bodies that we are *safe*. You are going to do this, not with words alone, but by slowly showing and proving to yourself that you are a person who is capable of influencing and choosing your life. You are going to do the most courageous thing imaginable and act against that fear—take it by the hand and say, *it's okay, you can stop protecting me, I love you, we're safe, watch me. . . .* The relationship with this voice doesn't have to be toxic forever. The more we take action against it, the more it starts to listen to us. The default voice that our minds fall back to will also change when *we* change. When we prove to it, with new behavior, that we are not the things it's trying to convince us we are, that voice in our head is eventually forced to change. It starts to see us as capable, resilient, full of joy and gratitude. It won't happen right away, it will take a lot of time. The old path won't go anywhere but it will become less frequented, no longer the highway of our minds, but a side path with weeds growing over it. It is no longer the easiest route—the one we have carved out intentionally for ourselves becomes the main path. Our old path can still be triggered up and visited out of habit, but it will slowly lose its power to affect the whole of us. We choose our own path, over and over, until it becomes the default route. And this is how we can begin to live differently, to live more freely, outside of the controlling limitations of our minds and that voice that seeks to keep us *small*.

YOU WERE ALWAYS HOLDING THE PEN, SO REWRITE YOUR STORY

You are not just the main character of your life; you are the fucking director, writer, stylist, casting director, and producer of it. You are in control of the allocation of your resources and where they go. Often, we just forget. Like, literally every fucking minute or so! Bringing our attention back to the pres-

YOU AREN'T JUST THE MAIN CHARACTER, YOU'RE THE FUCKING DIRECTOR!

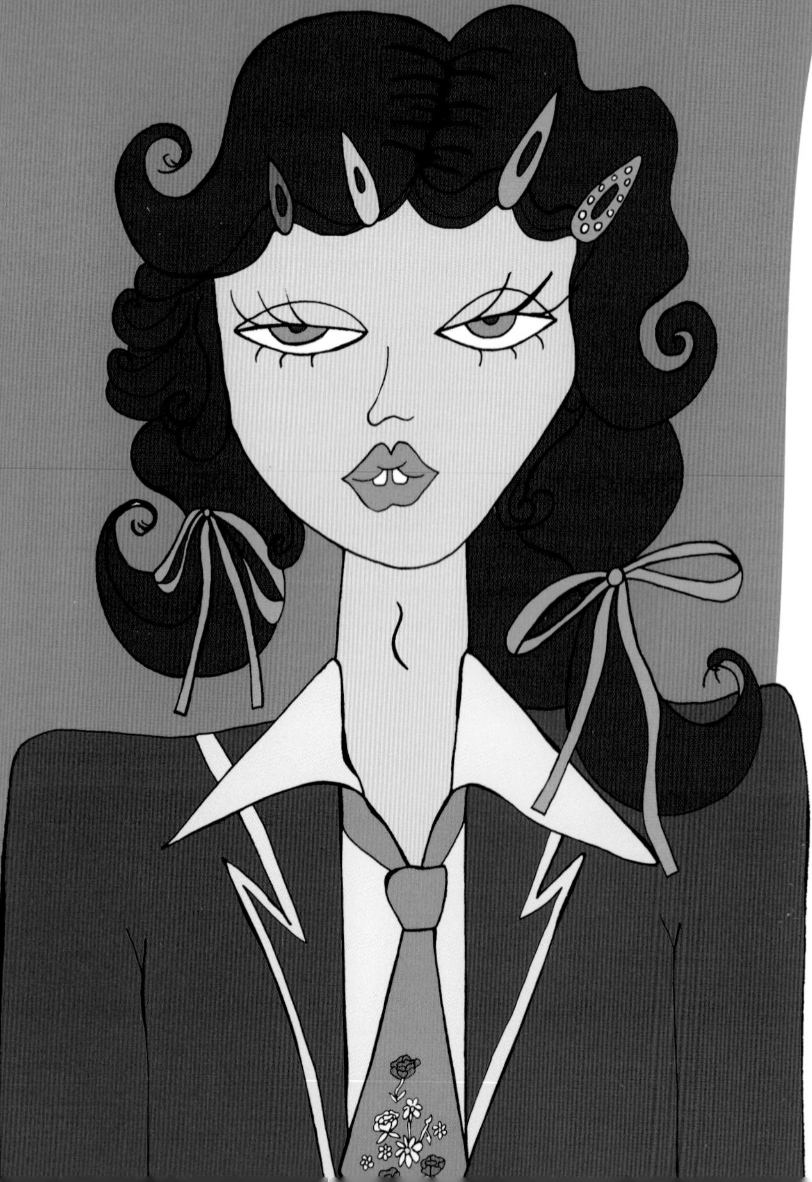

ent moment to make conscious and intentional choices is how we remind ourselves that we are in charge. This is how *we* can start to design our lives. Allowing nothing but the desires, the joy, the awe, the curiosity that has been buried beneath them the whole time to become the new and rightful architects of our life, in whatever shape or form that takes for you.

You can talk back to that fear and tell it not to dictate your life. Remind it you're in charge. That you do not desire to be small. Choose right now, say to that voice, *I am fine with making decisions that you do not agree with. I do not need you to understand me.*

I want you to be able to see the ways in which you outsource your own intuition. A parent's voice that lives in your head. An ex-partner's. A set of rules you strictly live by that cause you to feel shame when not abiding by them. To live delicious and fulfilling lives free of fear, resentment, and obligation, we need to create values of our own, values not dictated to us, but coming from WITHIN us. Neither feminism, patriarchy, your mate, nor your partner should tell you the values you should live your life by. Listen to yourself. Hold on to that truth. The answers are there.

Together, we're going to unpack how to tune out all the outside noise, recognize our own authority in determining our direction, and become our own fucking compass. For that, we need to examine those inner voices and how they manifest inside our minds. Let's take a look at what I like to call "the voice that lives in your head."

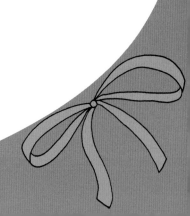

WHOSE VOICE IS IT ANYWAY?

We have 70,000 thoughts a day on average. A lot of them consist of the most absolute random *crap* you could possibly imagine. *I should get a pedicure done more often. Who's that wearing the big hat, they look important? Today is so shit. Mmmm, I thought this would taste better. I wonder how my Instagram post is doing?* The voice we hear from within, which won't stop talking and commenting on everything in life, has been the fascination of many philosophers and spiritual teachers for thousands of years. Everyone has a different name for it:

- Buddha called it the "monkey mind."
- Eckhart Tolle calls it the "ego."
- Dacher Keltner calls it "the default self."
- Most of us call it "me" or "my inner monologue."

This voice, the ego, is not just a mystical concept, but has a real location in our brains in a region known as the default mode network (DMN). Science has finally caught up with what ancient Eastern philosophers and Buddhists have known for millennia: that there is a part of the brain that won't shut up and that our ability to silence and distance ourselves from it can improve our quality of life.

This "voice" in our heads comes "online" and starts talking at us when we go "offline"—that is, when we are not focusing our attention on something. It's where our minds go when they "wander." It is essentially the autopilot setting of our brains. It comes on when we're not involved in a single-focused task. When we're doing something habitual that requires little attention—like driving, brushing our teeth—our attention goes back onto that inner voice. We might randomly remember some childhood friend we haven't spoken to for years while doing the dishes and they just suddenly appear in our mind, unprompted. *I wonder what so-and-so is up to?* We might even start having a heated argument with them in our head about something we don't even care about. One thought after the next, branching off the other and descending into chaos, hence Buddha's description of it as the "monkey mind." We come back online when we blink ourselves back into reality, realizing where our thoughts are going. It is not because "we" wanted to think about them at this moment in time but because our brain, out of habit, has defaulted to a set of thought patterns. Maybe we saw something that subconsciously triggered a memory of that friend and it stirred up an old set of thoughts. The same way our behaviors follow a pattern out of habit— taking our shoes off and putting the keys down when we get home from work without thinking about it—our thoughts have their own habitual patterns they perform on autopilot too. Our brains continue this stream of endless thoughts out of sheer habit, when we're not in the present moment and paying attention to the "now."

What do we hear when our "voice" gets triggered by certain stimuli in our environment? Let's say a woman in a red dress walks past and triggers thoughts of your first date with your partner, because you wore a red dress. Then you notice how great she looks in it. Then you spiral, remembering how you used to look in a red dress when you were younger. Then you compare yourself to her. Then you feel shit about yourself. And nothing has actually happened. Nothing. A woman walked past you in a red dress. If it was yellow, if you'd have taken a different route, you would not be feeling this way. But your attention followed your thoughts down a familiar path—uninterrupted—and now you feel like shit. If you do not interrupt this pattern by placing your attention onto something else, or separate yourself from this voice and develop an ability to talk back to it, or even laugh at it compassionately, it will possess you. It will take over your mood, you will *become* the voice instead of just watching it. You will

THE VOICE IN YOUR HEAD IS MAKING SUGGESTIONS NOT DEMANDS. YOU HAVE THE POWER TO IGNORE IT.

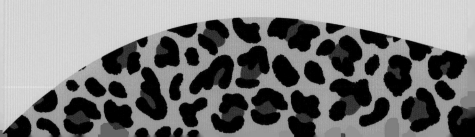

follow it down the rabbit hole and get trapped inside the mental loop of your thoughts and what you look like. It will disconnect you from the experience of being in your actual body.

SO HOW DO WE COME BACK ONLINE?

If this default voice only starts talking at us when we go offline—when we are not focusing on something_the way to escape this voice is to come back online as often as possible. The way to distance ourselves from the voice that talks at us all day is to gently bring ourselves back into the "now" by simply *noticing things.*

Mindfulness is the practice of bringing our attention back to the present moment. When we choose to focus on something in front of us—whether it is something beautiful, a smell, a taste, a texture, noticing the feeling of the shirt on our back, or even looking at a photo with the aim of silencing our thoughts—the "monkey mind" goes offline. We no longer hear the thoughts of the inner critic, the inner monologue, the constant running commentary of our minds that bring up the most random spewing of old events, arguments, someone's relationship we just saw on social media. This all gets silenced when we pay attention to the present moment as *that* now becomes our focus of attention.

I'm sure you can recall a moment when you experienced this brief "relief" from the inner voice. Perhaps when you felt the first rays of sunshine on your face in winter, the first beautiful sunset in a new city, the taste of new, delicious food you weren't expecting to be so good. For a brief second, the mind goes quiet. It is because you have shifted your attention from the part of your brain responsible for the running commentary of your life, that default mode network, onto something else. When your mind is absorbed fully by the moment, you become totally present, and you no longer need to listen to those thoughts.

The good news is, we don't have to wait for beauty to strike us, to be present and silence that voice. *We can consciously seek it out!* Paying attention to the beauty around us in our lives, such as the color of flowers, the texture of food while we eat, the feeling of a deep relaxing breath when our minds are going wild, is one way to bring our minds back online_remembering that we are in the driver's seat of where our attention goes. That we do get to choose our next move. That we can ignore the voice that is trying to keep us small.

The liberation from this bullying voice starts with simply noticing it and not following it down that path. It is the simple decision that the voice is not the dictator of our behavior. This is not easy. But when repeated enough times, we strengthen a new pathway. This is called "neuroplasticity"—our brains are able to adapt and change to develop new habits. Our behaviors are not set in stone, we have the power to change who we are. These new thoughts, when repeated, then become beliefs. Beliefs that shape and change our actions, which then become our habits and create the results we want.

For example, if our inner monologue starts to sound like this:

"Oh no, I missed my train! Fuck, why didn't I plan ahead properly? I've fucked everything up. This is so typical of—oh shit, okay, calm down."

Here! The moment when we REALIZE our minds are creating negative thoughts is when we can pause. Take a deep breath. And reframe it with curiosity:

"Okay, well, I'm sure something better is in store for me. Maybe there's someone on the next train I'm supposed to meet? Perhaps I'm being protected from something? There's nothing I can do about it, so I might as well accept it and hop around the station. What can I do with my time to fill it? Ah, there's a book I've wanted to read for months in the bookstore! Maybe this is leading to something better after all."

This is how we put a pin in our downward spiral and reach upward with curiosity, again and again. Soon, stressful situations become not obstacles

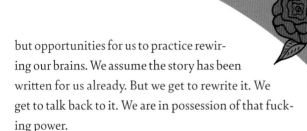

but opportunities for us to practice rewiring our brains. We assume the story has been written for us already. But we get to rewrite it. We get to talk back to it. We are in possession of that fucking power.

No, I am not a terrible human.

No, I am good enough to go out with my friends, and I'm going to the party.

No, I am worthy of love, as there are people who love me. I am going on that date.

No, I am hungry. I am going to eat.

No, I shouldn't leave, I deserve to be here. I am going to enjoy my meal at this fancy restaurant.

No, what I have to say is worth being heard. I am going to say it and feel the adrenaline of contributing to this conversation.

The moment we show the voice how much of a coward it is by acting against it, by bringing our attention back online, noticing something or taking a breath, the opportunity for more bliss and joy presents itself. We stop closing ourselves off from life, we feel confident from our successful attempts at ignoring the fear and we can begin to find and seek out joy fucking everywhere. We can even use the seeking of joy ITSELF as an intentional practice to silence this voice in our minds.

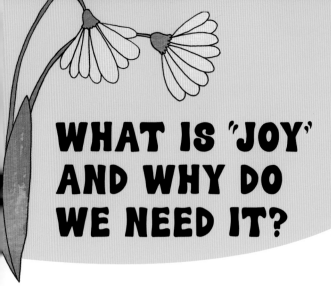

WHAT IS "JOY" AND WHY DO WE NEED IT?

Some call it "joy." Some call it "sacred." Some call it "awe." Some call it "bliss." Some call it "god." Some call it "the sublime." Some call it a "glimmer." Some call it "euphoria." Some call it . . ."*it.*" All these descriptions of joy have one thread in common: a sense of connection.

What I refer to as "joy" throughout this book isn't to be mistaken for a fleeting sensation of euphoria, happiness, ecstasy, or excitement (though joy is present in all of these emotions). Nor is it to be mistaken for the fake joy of a quick dopamine rush which later leaves us feeling depleted. The "joy" I am speaking of is a state of being. It is the delicious feeling of connection, curiosity, and wonder present in all human beings which lies behind that running commentary of the mind. It's a self-induced state of awe, a mental vacation from the neurotic, critical inner monologue of the "self," that can be brought on by intentionally relishing in the small pleasures of life.

This joy almost refuses to be defined—it is a peace and a contentedness, a feeling inside us that rises occasionally, perhaps when experiencing a warm encounter with a stranger or feeling delighted by a pleasure as small as the sun peeking out from behind a cloud on a gray day. It's the brief sense that we are connected to all things, delighted by what it feels like to be *alive in our bodies,* and temporarily forgetting how they look. When this joy is sustained for a longer period of time by immersing ourselves fully in an activity, psychologists call it being in a "flow state." It is the most blissful place for humans to exist, because this high has no hangover!

They say "time flies when you're having fun" for a reason—in this flow state, the area of our brains we use to calculate time in the prefrontal cortex shuts down. If you've ever blinked and found that hours have passed, you were likely in a delicious state of flow. These moments of embodied joy are so rare because our attention is all too often pulled in so many directions, the focus we require to remain in this state is hard to sustain. This is especially true for women, for whom the barrier to this feeling presents itself in a most insidious way. Women have been socialized to engage in every activity with a degree of awareness about what they look like *while* doing it. Many of us rarely get to step into this feeling of carefree joy because our mental resources are distracted by our appearance or our vigilance over our safety. It is impossible to fully "relax" into the present moment when there is always a degree of your attention outsourced onto how you *look* while you relax.

This is no fault of our own. Self-surveillance isn't a choice, it's a habit. We learn it is crucial for our survival to keep control over our appearance by not letting any unflattering parts of ourselves show, to avoid breaking the façade of perfection we are held to by society. This exists on a sliding scale. For some women it's an all-consuming burden that is carried into every single inter-action, watching for flaws in another's eyes. For some women it only flares up on days when they're feeling low and their view of themselves is tainted by the fog of depression. For some women, however, self-doubt is merely a thought that visits their mind but is no longer endorsed as true. That is the place we're aiming for. With lifelong, sustainable practice, it is possible for each and every one of us.

This is why seeking joy is so fucking important to reconnecting with our bodies, to unlearning the overwhelming self-obsession patriarchy demands of us. We have been trained since we were young to have our thoughts centered on our surveillance of our bodies, so much so that sometimes we notice little else; we lose our connection to the world and the people we inhabit it with. That fuzzy, euphoric, joyful connec-

tion from sustained attention gets intermittently blocked
by our awareness of our appearance.

Feeling and experiencing the world around us, seeking out moments of joy, is the way out of this self-conscious objectification. Maybe you feel "it" when the smell of coffee from a shop wafts so strongly past your nostrils, you stop to inhale it and feel a brief relief from the chatter in your mind that was nagging you for "eating so much." Or when a child smiles at you on the street. Or a sunset surprises you on your walk home. These moments, when joy grabs us and brings us into the here and now, remind us why life is worth living. They allow us to feel connected to the world around us. They pull us out of fear and into joy. They are how we learn to fall back in love with life, every time we forget and that magical veil is lifted, again and again and again.

This joy we feel in life's small pleasures is a moment of "awe." These moments might seem small on the surface, but don't dismiss them too quickly—they're more powerful than you think. They provide us a brief connection to the person we are behind our roles, our labels, the expectations others have of us. They temporarily extinguish that inner monologue, and with it, banish a great deal of the suffering we experience in our minds. In that moment we are able to just be.

The emotion of "awe" has been researched extensively by scientist Dacher Keltner. Any time I listen to him talk about the beauty of being alive, my eyes fill with tears! Keltner has proven with scientific research that what we are *feeling* in these beautiful moments intuitively has a physical basis. In the previous chapter we touched on the region of the brain called the default mode network—the network responsible for our inner monologue. *What's that over there? Oh you're looking a bit bloated today. I wonder how many steps it takes to walk to the moon?* It's no shock to hear that over-activity in this region of the brain, where our "voice" lives, is linked to an increased chance of depression. Through brain scans, Keltner discovered that this "self" region of the brain actually gets silenced (SILENCED!) in moments of awe. This brief "vanishing" of the inner critic, of our sense of "self," allows us to feel connected to the world around us, temporarily stopping our rumination and, therefore, our problems. In that moment, we don't exist. The "self" vanishes. We have no awareness of the past or future. These moments of awe and joy allow us to expand our consciousness from the narrow view of our "self" and experience a deeper connection to the world around us.

ARE YOU HEARING THIS? I need to check you fully understand how wild that is.

Awe isn't hard to find. We don't need to search far and wide to discover it, the trick is to train ourselves to find it in our everyday lives and to give it our attention—because IT IS ALL AROUND US. Keltner's research has found that experiencing these small moments, even for a few seconds a day, increases our life expectancy and helps reduce anxiety, stress, burnout, and depression. The more we connect to this part of ourselves, the more we experience the simple joy of being alive and the less we need external measures to make us feel seen or understood. We discover that these entry points into feeling joy and love are all around us. They are playing hide-and-seek. Waiting for us to uncover them. Keltner's scientific research on the effects of experiencing "awe" on the brain aligns with what spiritual leaders have been teaching intuitively for thousands of years. That when the mind quiets in appreciation of something beautiful, something inside us steps aside to allow us to feel a connection to something *bigger*. Better yet, this connection can be deepened if we fine-tune our minds to appreciate beauty, absolutely fucking everywhere.

DO THE SMALL THINGS REALLY BRING US JOY?

Every time the sun shines on my face it is as
though my anxious inner world melts
away. Suddenly I love everyone.
I can feel the cells

JOY IS ALWAYS SEEKING AN OPENING TO GUSH OUT!

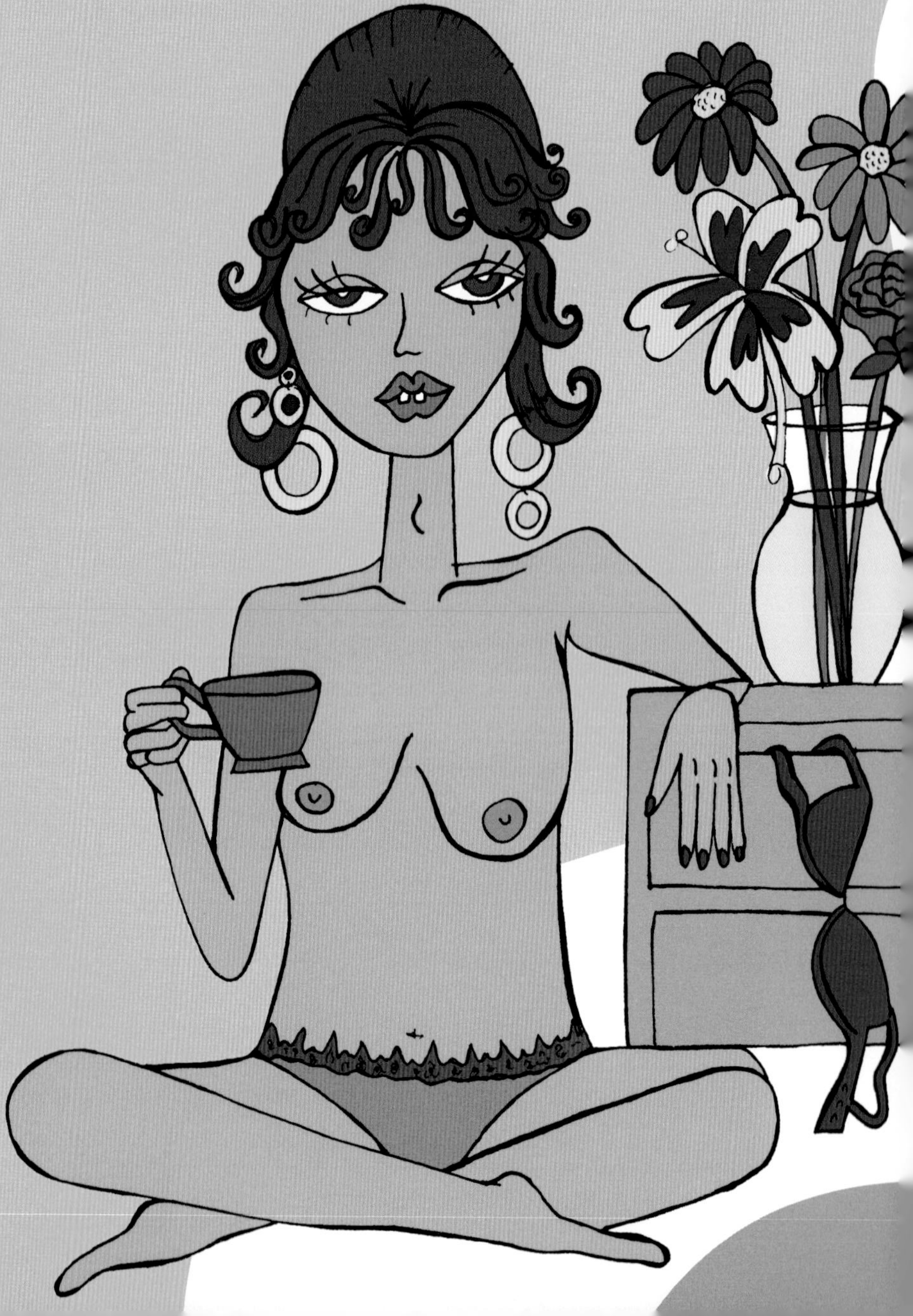

in my body waking up. I feel alive, delicious! I used to associate this feeling of aliveness and peace with *the sun*. I thought it was the sun that was *bringing* me joy. I thought the same of the other small pleasures in my life. I thought it was the flowers growing through the cracks in the pavements that *made* me feel delighted. The taste of the coffee in the morning that *made* me feel so alive. I thought it was the soft pillowy lips of the person kissing me that *gave* me joy.

I was once reading *The Power of Now* by Eckhart Tolle and I paused in awe on the line: "Joy can only exist when there is a gap in the stream of your thoughts."

The small things do not "give" us joy. What the sun, the flowers, the coffee, and people's lips do is create "a gap in our thoughts" through the sheer force of their beauty. By silencing the mind, the joy inside is no longer blocked. It is free to pour OUT! Only when we are open, can the light visit us.

This explains why life felt so "flat" when I was depressed or anxious. Why I could not be present for sex at times, missing out on the pleasure of the experience because the voice in my mind wouldn't shut up about how awkward my body looked in a certain position. The light, the joy, the delight, could not get through that mental cloud. There was no "gap" for the sun to shine! The beauty of these things—the sun, a song that moves us to tears, the smell of fresh bread—they catch the attention of our senses and YANK us back to the present moment, out of our heads and *into* our bodies. The connection we feel in these moments of life was always there—just like the sun behind the clouds.

The habit of seeking beauty is one small and radical practice we can use to reverse the self-conscious gaze that has pestered us our whole lives, focusing on our image. We reverse it by asking, "What in the world delights me?" instead of, "Do I look delightful enough for the world?"—no longer a woman that seeks to be looked at, but a woman that seeks to look at things!

STOP WAITING, START SEEKING

When I realized this, I no longer had to wait for beauty to visit me, or to be delighted , all I had to do was pay attention to the world, allow myself to be enraptured by it, allow it to steal my attention away from my appearance or the voice in my mind. In these moments, my body is not an obstacle to my joy, she is fucking *perfect!* She is doing exactly what she was fucking created to do—allowing me *to feel.* In these moments, I go from merely "knowing" intellectually that my body doesn't exist to be pretty, to FEELING that I am more than my body. In these moments, my body is not something that needs hiding, covering, sucking in, something that requires perfecting—it is a beautiful physical form, built for me to experience whatever life has to offer me in the present moment. For a second, there is no resistance or irritation, but complete surrender. I'm not "unworthy." I'm not a "bad friend." I'm not "unproductive." I'm not even a "woman." I'm a ball of fire and energy that wants to find something to spark with!

The joy comes from within. It has been resting inside all of us, waiting for an opening, waiting for us to acknowledge it and bring it back to life. When we pay attention and slow down, we awaken it. The trouble is we need to be "open" to allow these things to delight us, and our joy gets constantly blocked by our thoughts, it gets blocked by the layers of shame, cultural messaging, trauma, and fear that remain unhealed inside us, clouding our minds. We need to be "open" to allow the joy in.

I decided that I would not wait for these joyous moments to be presented to me. I would not wait for the perfect conditions to spontaneously arise in my life to permit myself to feel this way: wait to lose weight to enjoy the beach, wait to like my body to have the best shag of my life, wait until I had the "time" to go for a walk and bask in the sun. Instead, I would intentionally seek out and create these moments wherever I could, to integrate them into my days, to use them as tools to create an opening and to feel that sense of aliveness inside me, whether I "believed" I deserved that feeling or not. I had connected to something beautiful within me that could not be taken, in an otherwise fragile and impermanent world. My connection to this "joy" didn't mean I would never experience that fearful voice, or insecurities, but that they were no longer running the show. This was the beginning of claiming back the playful, curious sense of wonder I thought I had lost forever. The way out of my darkness was not to leap unrealistically into a state of pleasure and happiness, but to inch closer towards it, one curious question, one small experience at a time.

I have often been asked, "How are you so happy and confident?" It wasn't something I could ever articulate or answer *until* I lost it. Until my connection to this joy vanished, when I started to listen to that voice of fear in my head as though it was the truth. I had to find answers from the bottom of a dark hole I wasn't sure I would ever escape. I had become so resentful and irritated by everything in the world around me, overwhelmed by the fog of my mind, I wasn't sure if there was anything worth living for. Basic self-care like taking a shower was a burden. I knew deep down that no one was coming to save me. I had to learn how to fall in love with life all over again, picking up the practices I had slowly started to abandon. This time, with the power of doing them *intentionally*.

Seeking joy is not frivolous. It is not silly. I realized from the bottom of that hole that it's not something that I could wait for *it* to happen *to me*. That I could no longer afford the romance and joy of my life to be an afterthought, the icing, or the decoration. The romance and joy of my life had to be baked into the fucking cake from scratch.

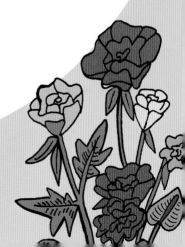

YOUR JOY IS CONTAGIOUS

I knew I had to write this book when, after sharing my small pleasures online, I received messages from women asking me, "But how can I feel joy without guilt?"

Guilt is one of the other barriers we experience when it comes to accessing our joy because, well, it makes you feel fucking terrible for having it! It's another form of shrinking. Of staying *small* because we don't want to attract envy, or people accusing us of being selfish. When we're socialized to be selfless good girls, which most women are, our own personal joy, our desire to bloom and expand may feel like we're being selfish, like we're being *bad girls*. And unfortunately, NOT in the hot kinky way! But feeling joy is not a barrier to being a good person, it is the enabler of it. The catalyst. Since I have noticed the fruits of my own joy, by prioritizing my pleasure at the center of my life, I can no longer ignore how contagious this joy is. I have watched how my joy has impacted not just my life, but my relationships and even the strangers I now have more patience and kindness for. Your joy and relaxation is not "selfish," because it also belongs to every single person you share your life with. Even if it's someone in traffic or the person serving you coffee. Your joy and relaxation affords you this inner spaciousness that allows you to choose to be kinder. You need to trust that you will have more to give, from a full cup. It is generous for you to love the shit out of your life. Where has pleasing others out of exhaustion got you?

When we choose ourselves instead of pleasing others, we become less resentful. The joy and energy I cultivate for myself by saying "NO" to things I'm uncomfortable with, don't want to do, or don't have time for, creates a pool of potent energy that spills over into everything around me. Joy is inherently selfless because joy is a fucking contagion. It is impossible to gatekeep and hoard, it is a light that shines out of us and onto everything around us. I had never considered that taking care of my needs and setting boundaries would enable me to give more generously to others—in a much more focused and intentional way—than when I had been exhausting myself for them. Setting boundaries feels the opposite of being a "giving" person. But joy is not selfish, it is the prerequisite to bringing the most kind, compassionate, and selfless version of yourself to the table. Joy provides us the bandwidth for generosity. To give from a place of abundance, instead of obligation.

The skip in your step, your increased levels of alertness, and energy alone will have a positive impact on others. Another study carried out by Dacher Keltner revealed people were more likely to help a stranger if they had gazed mindfully at a tree for two minutes, rather than at a building. Filling ourselves with wonder and awe in life enables us to feel more responsibility and compassion towards others, as we experience a deeper connection to the world through paying attention to it. A life of inner wealth and abundance allows the excess to spill over, feeding, fueling, and fertilizing everything around it.

This question I so often get asked—"How can I feel joy without guilt?"—stems from many of us falsely believing that joy operates within a capitalist framework, as though it is some scarce resource and to be in possession of it is to take something from someone else. But joy is not a zero-sum game. It is a state of being you create for yourself. Most of us have been sold a skewed idea of joy as something obtained from material possessions, so we keep reaching outside ourselves to spend money chasing it. Yet if we look at our actual experience, most of us can recall many times when we have been somewhere fancy, wearing something trendy—and still felt intensely miserable. On the opposite side of the spectrum, we've had moments when everything was going absolutely tits up and yet we somehow found existential joy and laughter in such a chaotic event. That is because joy is a state of *being*. Joy belongs to the realm of *feeling*. Of being connected. It is the surprise of it that can delight us! It's in our instinctual reaction to turn towards the sun when it peeks out, the fizz we feel in our bodies when we make eye contact with someone after laughing, the connection we feel when a beautiful sentence describes the way we have always seen the world, but never been able to express. This surprise is delightful, because even though we may be feeling terrible, anxious, or stressed, something beautiful has taken an axe to our layers of defense, creating a crack that opens and inspires a laugh or a smile, reminding us that we aren't completely frozen over. The relief that there is still joy there beneath us is a form of joy in itself.

Could you imagine if we all remembered this power of connection? To be delighted by life in this way? Capitalism wouldn't have a fucking leg to stand on! No longer would people be able to coerce you into relationships with bare minimum treatment. No longer would your image be the focal point of your existence. We would stop reaching out and buying as much stuff, spending and being on the hedonic treadmill of life, chasing achievement

IT IS GENEROUS FOR YOU TO LOVE THE SHIT OUT OF YOUR LIFE!

after achievement,
one after the other, being miserable in between hoping the next one will
pay off. We're taught this delight exists outside us,
but it's not. It's within us.

I write all of this not to confirm and validate the beliefs of
individuals whose world view centers around their own pleasures
at the expense of others, but for women like me, who have found themselves riddled with guilt about experiencing joy and love and laughter, or even
struggle to justify that they deserve it with their life full of responsibilities.
The women who write to me and say they feel guilty for buying themselves
something, lose sleep over unanswered messages, or feel torn between choosing the *guilt* of canceling a plan, or the *stress* of attending it when they don't
have the energy.

I want you to know that to fall madly in love with your life by designing
it to align with your pleasure, to relish every moment, to feel it all, to live authentically, is an immensely generous contribution you can give to the planet
and the people around you. To live authentically is to receive the gift of your
unique and unrepeatable life with gratitude, giving others the courage and
permission to do the same for themselves. Your authenticity and the joy that
emanates from it is a gift.

It's time to squeeze out every ounce and gorge on the delicious feast that
life has all around us. Your joy is not selfish. It is a generous gift to this planet,
like a little light that flickers on the globe, slowly brightening it up, one light
bulb at a time. Your joy is not selfish, how could it be when it courses through
you, radiating out of your every pore, giving others the courage to step out of
their own darkness?

MIND THE GAP!

What does it say that I feel most alive when my phone is *dead*?

Your attention is so powerful (thank you VERY much for giving it to me), and it is one of your most valuable resources. Everyone and everything is competing for it. From social media, to the latest TV show, your job, every store on the street, every label in the supermarket, the new stretch marks on your legs, the negative scenarios you replay in your head, everything and everybody wants a slice of your awareness and attention.

So how do we decide where to place our focus? Whatever we decide to give our attention to has our power. We give it our energy. Our attention can be used to be present and still, allowing our minds to experience moments of peace, inspiration, and calm, to seek out beauty in the world. But the problem is that we're all so busy, we rarely get to consciously "choose" where our attention is placed unless we make *pausing* an intentional habit. Unless we create "gaps" they're going to be taken away from us once more. Before we have time to consider, we've been fast tracked onto the next thing. No time to pause. Contemplate. Change our minds. Stop.

The mental gaps we have between Zoom meetings, TV episodes, online videos, dating apps, and lunch breaks are all becoming increasingly colonized by "the next thing to do." There is very little room for our minds to wander or be bored since there is always something to focus our attention on next. There is barely any room for original thought to be born and expose itself, because we are already being ushered onto the next moment. The next task. The next thing we need to do in our lives.

Capitalism has designed our lives in a way that we are never ever satisfied, so we constantly reach outside ourselves for more. Making us "satisfied" has never been its goal, instead it wants to keep us hungry. To rely on the insatiable wanting of our ego, which seeks to boost itself with material possessions to gain love, praise, or attention. Having to come back for more and more and more. Phones break quickly so we buy a new one. Trends cycle in and out every week ensuring we're always behind. Our clothes are made poorly, so we buy more. Social media algorithms are deliberately unpredictable so we keep posting, keep doing things we don't actively want to for more likes in the clothes we don't like, uploaded by the phone that will soon break. As long as nothing is ever "enough" we will always be good consumers, reaching outside ourselves, filling every moment of our lives trying to feel something.

Consider the gaps that appear in our days: while we walk on the pavement, waiting at the bus stop, a silence in conversation, a ride in an elevator with someone, between two tasks, as we wait for a kettle to boil, a microwave to ping, right now before you read the next sentence . . . In these invisible spaces, we can either get out our phones, find a new distraction, or we can choose to be present. Being present and staying in the "boredom" without numbing ourselves is where ALL the good shit happens, this is the space in our lives for realizations we've been avoiding. To realize "that didn't feel right" or to finally discover the idea for a creative project we've been waiting for. The space to lock eyes with someone we would have missed if we were looking into our screens. Or to ponder a new perspective on a building we walk past every day. To choose differently. To avoid logging onto Instagram and ruining our day by obsessing over people's lives we constantly compare ourselves to. We have been trained to think "the next thing" has more importance, more pleasure, than where we are right here, right now. The "fake fun" of a quick dopamine hit reduces our ability to appreciate the small moments of beauty in life. We become numb to the subtle flavors of the world around us and require more and more regular hits. It erodes our connection to intuition. We get hooked on short-term fixes. This is why we are encouraged to constantly be "on" as it keeps us distracted, it is why women are taught to focus so much on their image that at times we can't think about anything else, collecting

WHAT KIND OF
BEAUTIFUL IDEAS
RUSH IN WHEN
YOU LEAVE THE
GAPS OF YOUR MIND
OPEN WITHOUT
FILLING THEM?

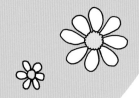

a graveyard of experiences in which we were physically present, but not *mentally* there. We are being taught to outsource our intuition into external things instead of within ourselves, and the same too with our attention. The little gaps within our lives, these small moments, are where we can start to claim back our time and create more spaciousness, more room to *choose* where our attention is spent.

- A walk in the park without your phone is a gap.
- Taking one long, deep breath is a gap.
- Noticing the rose shrub next to you at the bus stop instead of taking a photo of it is a gap.
- Making your coffee and focusing on each step is a gap.
- Listening to the world's chatter around you is a gap.
- Allowing the plane in the sky to distract you from your thoughts is a gap.
- Counting the freckles on the face of your lover is a gap.
- Walking on the sunny side of the street and relishing in the sensation of the sun soaking into your pores is a gap.
- Watching the world move by on a train rather than scrolling mind-numbingly on social media is a gap.
- Waking up and opening the window to get some fresh air rather than reaching for your phone is a gap.
- Sitting in the space between one meeting and the next is a gap.

These small moments may not seem big, but they are slowly being stolen from us and utilized without our resistance. We replace these moments of "boredom" that would previously have allowed our minds to wander or engage in conversation with a stranger, with the most instant dopamine-inducing thing, usually whacking out our phones to fill the silence. This is by no means judgmental. We all do it, the addiction is part of the design, but that doesn't mean we shouldn't try to examine why we do it and what we miss out on. We need to look at the cost.

Because what we choose to give our attention to dictates our experience of life. Think of the last time you finished watching a TV episode, and before you were given a moment to consider whether you wanted to watch the next one a little countdown began telling you it was about to start. Before you know it, you've rolled onto the next one, given no time to think, *I should stop now and go to bed to get a good night of sleep!* The attention economy jumps in and overrides our decision-making. We binge the series even though we planned to watch just one episode, go to sleep four hours later than we wanted. We wake up later; with little sleep we're more reactive and so we might snap at our partner, a co-worker, or friend.

So even though these gaps appear inconsequential, the stripping away of our decision-making capacity greatly impacts our lives. Because having the space to reflect, to ask ourselves *What do I want?*, gives us the emotional bandwidth to be able to respond, instead of just reacting to our environment. Filling our minds with content removes that possibility.

The goal is to consciously pause, check in, breathe, and create space in our lives where there isn't any, to ensure the next decision is made with intention. This is how we can claim our lives back one moment at a time.

If we try to allow joy to arise in the smallest of pleasures, we develop minds that are strengthened against the ploys of advertising, splurging, and chasing. If we create lives that we don't *need* a holiday from, because we find pauses for relaxation whenever possible, we become less of a compliant consumer. And, yes, we are freer. We become an active player in the pursuit of our joy instead of waiting for it to be delivered to us in these intense, hedonistic chunks. We no longer need to fill and fill and fill ourselves with content—things, thoughts, clutter. We become the source of joy, of play, of the ability to allow our minds to roam, wander, and create as we did naturally when we were kids. Making up stories, creating little worlds, and asking curious, original questions.

Increasing these gaps in our lives is hard, as there is a demanding distraction at every turn. Even writing this chapter, I have fought and lost the urge to search "pink butter dishes" because I saw one online. Consumerism has convinced us all that happiness is one purchase away. Often we are not buying the product, we are buying into the version of ourselves we imagine we will *become* when we buy it. When other people see we have it, it is another badge on our public image which signals something to others about "who we are," or who we *want* them to think we are. When we use products or even *people* as a vehicle of proving ourselves or seeking to create an identity, we suffer. After the initial high of the purchase, the car, the house, the relationship we thought would complete us, we return to the baseline of despair and the void appears once more. Now the void wants something *bigger*. Its stomach has stretched, its appetite has grown, and it needs more and more to satiate it.

Distraction is everywhere, and it's an ongoing journey of bringing our minds back to what we're doing in the present moment, to be able to design our lives more consciously. It's a practice and something we will have to return to for the rest of our lives. But we need to intentionally choose to try. To stop running. Avoiding. Numbing. We need to choose to see what life has to say to us in those gaps. We need to slow down.

If chosen time and time again, this practice becomes a habit. And the best part is, it's free, accessible, and we don't have to meditate in a field to achieve it. It might sound overwhelming, the idea of being "conscious" of everything we do, but that is not the aim. We just need a few seconds, at random times in the day, to bring our minds back to the present. Through this, we can start to notice just how addicted we are to dopamine distractions. How many times our arms reach for our phones in a moment of boredom. When I first started to notice this, it was alarming as fuck! But we cannot change what we are not aware of. Awareness is beautiful.

Somewhere along the way, we forgot that we could fucking choose. We're not striving to become perfectly happy, or constantly present, but aiming to create more space between our authentic nature and our default programming. Only then can we begin to discover and reconnect to our joy, to what truly makes us happy. It is waiting for us, in those gaps.

All we need to do is learn to say "NO."

NO.

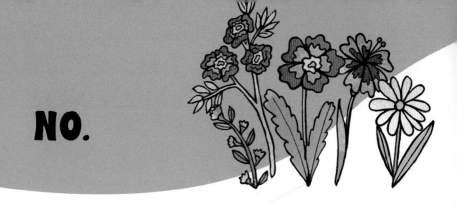

I had an alternative title in mind for this book a few years ago. I was going to call it *NO*. Not, *The Power of No* or *The Art of Saying No* or *How to Say No*. Too much explaining! Simply, *NO*.

The key to creating more room for joy in our lives is "NO." It is a word I wish women had ready loaded at the forefront of their brains, instead of shoved right at the back, brought out only in extreme circumstances and, in my experience, even *then* struggling to be mustered. We respond habitually instead with: *"Yes, I can squeeze that in the diary! Yes, my week's a bit packed and I haven't had much sleep, but yes I can make it! Yes yes yes!"* Enough squeezing! Enough packing in! "NO" is a word quite foreign on the tongues of women who believe that having "limits" makes them selfish. Saying "NO" goes against our training to be small, agreeable, and likeable. But those of us who feel they cannot say "NO" are ticking time bombs, waiting for just enough pressure for the bitterness, overwhelm, and resentment of our unmet needs to explode. Saying "NO" helps us to relieve this build-up of pressure in the first place. It prevents us from becoming Women Living Exhaustedly!

Once we learn how to use this "NO" we can liberate ourselves from the mental shackles of constantly proving, pleasing, perfecting—and step into a life we have actively designed for ourselves, full of "FUCK YES" and "FUCK NO" instead of "Sure" and "Ummmmmm okay, that's fine." And if there's anything we do find that we are uncertain of, we can say "NO" by stating that we need more time to think.

In order to live lives driven by our intentional design, instead of from a place of fear and resentment, we must reclaim "NO"—and the delicious spaciousness that "NO" opens up for us. Suddenly, there is more room than we

YOUR BOUNDARIES AREN'T SUPPOSED TO BE CONVENIENT.

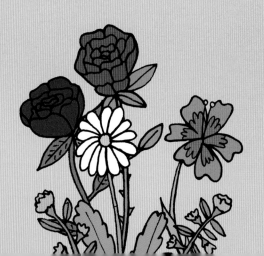

had before, when we were filling it with the needs of others. "NO" is going to afford you the space to gain perspective in life. Whether that means closing the door to your bedroom for privacy. Telling someone you need time to think before making a decision. Turning off the TV to get a good night's sleep. Rescheduling a plan you don't have the time for. "NO" is how you claim back the precious resource of your energy and attention that you have been passively and unconsciously siphoning out of yourself. "NO" is the patch you use to cover up those holes where energy has been leaking out.

"NO" is a word that was not in my vocabulary for years. My "good girl" training kept me agreeing to things I didn't want to do while the resentment piled higher and higher in the background. I wanted to be seen as strong and capable of handling anything. The fear of letting people down kept me agreeing to things I couldn't commit to. The irony of this, of course, was that I constantly let people down *because* I was spreading myself too thinly. Pleasing became its own prison, because my ego could never admit that my workload was too much for me to handle, and so I never took the rest I needed. My perfectionism was calling the shots, it had me afraid that if I just slowed down, I wouldn't be enough without the proving, chasing, and hustling. Every time I said "yes" to something I didn't want to do, I drove myself further from the life I desired, and closer to resentment and burnout.

By developing a relationship with "NO" and, by default, an acceptance of my own mental and physical limitations, I began to create the space I needed to look at my life from a calm, still place and assess where the hell I was going and, most importantly, *why*. We need to create space in our lives for joy. It can't find us when we're running, numbing, perfecting, chasing, hustling, stressing ourselves into the ground. "NO" is freedom. Saying "NO" to something means saying "YES" to ourselves.

NO...

That timing doesn't work for me.

I don't have the room to take this on.

I'm not comfortable with you showing up without texting first.

I need you to knock before entering please.

I'm not comfortable discussing this at the moment.

No, thank you.

No, that's not who I am.

No, it's my turn to speak.

No, I can't.

No.

No.

No.

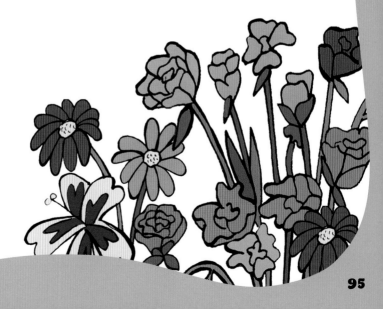

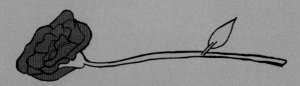

YOUR REST IS YOUR RESPONSIBILITY

Saying "NO" opens up a precious gap in our lives. I like to view a bench in a public space as a physical gap. A gentle suggestion for rest, patiently dwelling among the buildings that demand our busyness, time, money, labor, among the spaces that ask us to consume something to exist in public. A public bench doesn't ask you to *do* anything, it suggests you can just *be*. Park benches in particular have been my own personal altars for healing and stillness. They are their own "NO" in the middle of the city.

Eckhart Tolle calls the things that calm us down and bring us into the moment "portals to the present." Isn't that magical? His most frequently used example of an accessible "portal" is taking one conscious deep breath. In focusing on taking one conscious breath, it is impossible for the mind to think about anything else. Your brain can only think of one thing at a time, so in focusing on your breath your thoughts temporarily come to a halt. Taking a breath is a "NO" to our spiraling thoughts.

I've observed how gaps manifest in urban spaces, too. Not just benches, but a bistro set, a stoop, a nook, an archway, a ledge, a park itself is a gap—they all act as carved-out spaces in the world for us to pause, enjoy a view, or rest. Each provides a retreat from the chaos of our inner and outer lives, encouraging us to perch, sit, ponder, relish—do nothing, say "NO" to the hyper-acceleration in and around us. It is beautiful to me that even in the physical world, humans erect altars that respect the need for rest. Especially in today's world, their very existence seems deliciously radical. We need to find these areas of rest within ourselves, too. In her book *How to Do Nothing*, Jenny Odell talks of how her favorite rose garden was once almost converted into a block of condos; she then writes, "I see a similar battle playing out for our time, a colonization of the self by capitalist ideas of productivity and efficiency. One might say the parks and libraries of our selves are always about to be turned into condos."

The gaps in our minds are also being taken over. Without our resistance. Without protest. But unlike a library or a rose garden, we cannot demonstrate in front of them, protesting their demolition. These precious gaps are being manipulated by social media's insatiable appetite for our focus, energy, and spare time, and our only form of protest is to withdraw our attention. If you're one of the 93 percent of people who take their phone to the toilet, you are not alone. Tech has taken over our fucking lives! Gaps and opportunities for mental rest and reset are everywhere, but they are being colonized by capitalism and tech, exploiting our most valuable commodity—our attention.

City spaces are now even designed with fewer benches to optimize the time it takes us to get from one money-spending zone to the next. We're not encouraged to dwell. Some benches are now designed to be uncomfortable so we don't spend too long there. This is part of a wider movement called "hostile architecture" in which the aim is to prevent homeless people from sleeping on benches, kids skateboarding on them, or anyone loitering too long. It actively discourages many people from participating in public space at all. *Where the fuck are we all supposed to hang out?*

Social media has by default become our new "mall," where we all go to collectively hang out. It also uses the same hostile design: with no breaks in its content, we spend longer absorbed by it and are more likely to buy things from it. Sure, social media is free, but our attention is the currency these platforms trade in to keep running. Think of their interface as being like a mall or a public space where

GET QUIET FOR A LITTLE WHILE AND SEE WHAT COMES THROUGH...

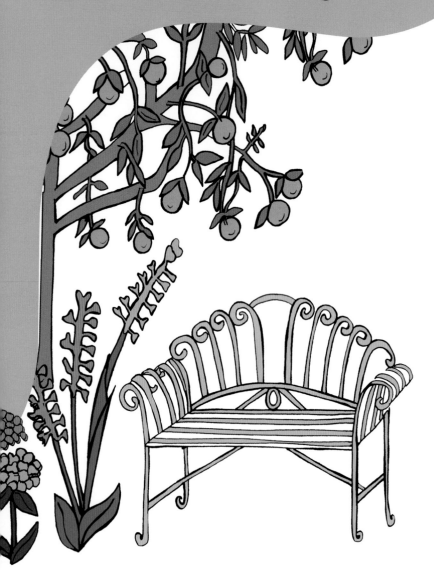

spending is encouraged, keeping us moving with no space to rest, no benches, unless we spend money. This is why public benches are radical, they ask for nothing in return but that you be still, in deep contemplation with them.

MENTAL BENCHES

Our minds are like parks. Without a mental bench to sit on for a moment of pause, we create no space to peacefully observe the goings on, to choose which path we want to walk down and what decision we should take next. All too often we push on, we keep running the same route without pause because there is always an endless surplus of things to do, stuff to buy, emails to send, something to fix—our "rest" is dismissed entirely, never considered, as we're shuttled from one productive task to the next. This is how most of us are encouraged to spend our lives, saving our rest for some day in the future when we hope it will be easier. There are multiple ways we dismiss joy and play from our life—I will enjoy fashion *when* I lose weight. I will be happy *once* I receive a promotion. I will get eight hours of sleep *once* this job is over. I will feel whole *when* my ex realizes they made a mistake. But to always delay joy and rest for the future is to glaze over our entire lives, discounting that *these* days also count, dismissing what we have right now and holding out for a mythical "happy ever after" which may never fully arrive. We can't afford to keep delaying rest. It does not have to be something grand, it can be small. We need to carve out mental "benches" for rest in our lives the way they were erected in cities, even if it is only for a single minute a day. We need space to think, to collect ourselves, to check in with our bodies.

These gaps are necessary in every area of our lives. Eckhart Tolle says that the frequency of the "gaps" between even each thought, determines our quality of life. So, if the frequency of the gaps in our stream of thoughts— uncolonized by productivity or chasing the next high—determines our ability to enjoy life, it makes sense that almost every behaviour modern culture encourages us to do, was built to distract us from them. When we are robbed of stillness we never have a moment to consult ourselves, to uncover how to use "NO." Because those moments of stillness, like a bench in a busy city or a moment of reflection before we go to buy something, pose a threat to our consumer habits and impulse choices. The choices we make driven by the fear of missing out and the urgency we feel in an environment where slowing down doesn't seem like an option. If we slowed down a little, turned our phones off, closed social media, and went for a walk, we may discover the urgency was false. We might realize there is nothing to miss out on after all. We might spend less money. We might stop outsourcing our power.

Our attention *is* the product, and they need it! Benches in the world and in the mind need to be protected. They create opportunities for a pause, allowing us the space required for more conscious decision-making from a place of clarity and abundance. The way we guard these gaps is with a "NO" to our attention continuously being distracted.

YOUR REST IS YOUR RESPONSIBILITY

One thing I know for sure, is that the body will always whisper to us when she's tired. She will always tell us when we need a break, through a yawn, back pain, or perhaps sickness. Even when we keep taking in more and more content and more stimulus, our bodies remind us of our limits.

When I was burnt out, I did not have any gaps to pause. It was all about moving forwards, proving myself, and never stopping. *Proving what?* you ask. *God knows!* The answer to that question would only reveal itself to me once I slowed down and paused long enough for the pain, the hurt, the perfectionism, and the unhealed wounds to rise up so that I could observe them, no longer outrunning the pain. It's hard to recognize unhealthy coping mechanisms when they're praised, when workaholism literally makes you successful. Even when the life you have created starts to feel like an exhausting performance, if it receives love and praise, why *would* you be motivated to dismantle it?

I tried to be the perfect activist, feminist, writer, boss, daughter, friend, lover, woman as though it would protect me from being abandoned or criticized. If I could get everything right, please everyone, I could avoid feeling unworthy—so I believed. We are convinced that with just enough pleasing, with just enough things ticked off our lists, with just enough beauty, with just enough proving, with just enough striving, we can become enough—and only *then* will we be able to finally experience peace. But perfection is not protection. It will not protect you from people not liking you. It will not protect you from people leaving you. All my time was spent proving I could do it all. I had always been ambitious, but a lot of it was being subconsciously driven by fear. *"Floss will get it done, she always does!"* is something that someone has actually said about me in the middle of a meeting about whether or not a very tight deadline I had was manageable. After feeling the initial intense frustration at this person, I realized it was not *their* fault that they thought this, this was the set up I had created around me. This was the expectation I had forged in the minds of others because I had never said "NO" to work. *I had allowed this to happen.* I was not the "victim" of my busyness, but the architect of it!

I had learned from a young age, as a lot of women do, to strive for perfection to receive love. It was me who still had unrealistic expectations of myself and so tirelessly tried to prove myself with larger-than-life ambition. The people in my life had never actually heard me say "NO," because there was a voice in my head that told me *leisure and rest is for the weak.* Can you relate to this voice? That internal side-eye you feel before you can even think about saying "NO" to taking something else on? Are you critical of others *around you* who aren't as productive?

Just as a woman doesn't need to be told directly that she is ugly to criticize herself in the privacy of her bedroom mirror, because she has internalized the critical voice, I too would act as my own surveillance camera, monitoring whether I was at peak productivity. As if at any moment that I dared to rest someone would run out and say, *"gotcha, you're weak!"* My attempts at relaxation were pathetic! I would take my laptop into the bath and turn it into a brainstorming session. Or edit my videos on a walk to the grocery store. I was never present, productivity had colonized even my rest. When our "doing" is fueled by a desire to prove something, avoid something, it won't be long until the friction of going full speed without rest causes us to burn out. We are not machines . . . and even machines need fucking oiling. The gaps in our lives are the lubrication we need to not turn into fucking robots! Those gaps, when our nervous system is relaxed, provide the space for healing to occur in the stress-induced body.

It wasn't until I had a physical illness that I gave myself permission to rest. I was lucky, because I was then able to rest and mend and I felt assured that no one could call me "weak." *It was my body! It wasn't my fault!* But, of course, it was my fucking fault. I was the one who pushed myself to that point in the first place. I had ignored the whispers from my body. I believe, now, that part of me wanted to burn out so I could point to my body as the "reason" for needing rest. Not "me." Admitting I needed to slow down felt far too vulnerable. I once tried to go into the studio to record a podcast episode with a bag of frozen peas wrapped around my hip and another in the small of my back, screaming in agony any time I lifted my arms, because there was an electric shock going down my leg from a slipped disc. My ambition was bigger than me. It always has been. But this was deeper than ambition. I was outrunning my fear of not being good enough. I wish I could give that version of myself a hug, but since I can't, I am begging you to give *yourself* a permission slip to rest. Because no one is going to fucking give it to you. We need to be the ones to say "NO."

GUARDING YOUR GAPS

I realized that I didn't need to quit my work altogether, drop my responsibilities, or reject consumerism entirely to heal from my relentless people-pleasing. What I needed was to *integrate* rest into my life, to carve it out and protect it as much as I did with work. A gap is available to everyone. Even just a breath, listening to birds while you make coffee, pausing before walking through a doorway. You are doing the same things, *but simply adjusting your state of being while you do them.* The direction we are heading in does not have to be dictated to us, we can design it—but only if we stop.

When our lives are lived on default for too long without any pause to consider whether our

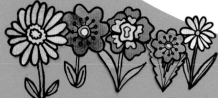

desires have changed, we can feel great friction and resistance in our everyday lives. It is because we are performing an expired role. We need to take a peek behind the curtain and check in with ourselves, to step back from those roles and remember the vibrant joy and life of the person behind them. Personally, early mornings have become the time of the day that I've carved out for my "self-peeking." And I mean CARVED out, rather than accidentally stumbled upon. Because when we create time to connect with ourselves, we can enter our roles fully, with the fresh perspective to redesign and tailor them to fit us better. Let's try to hear the whisper before the scream.

LIFE WITH NO GAPS

When I visited Tokyo, I saw people collapsing on floors, falling asleep on pavements and on top of cars in their pristine black work suits on a Saturday morning, having stayed out after their shift at work. Just like many places in the world, the weekend offered a way to escape the pressures and demands of their working life, and were typically reserved for indulging in excess. This is known locally as a Shibuya meltdown and the Japanese even have a word—*karoshi* 過労死)—which literally translates as "overwork death." It describes a sudden death caused by working so many hours a week that the stress brings on a stroke or heart attack, or because a person ends their life instead of going back to the pressures of work. Many workers have died by suicide after logging over one hundred hours monthly overtime, and in 2018 the government responded by capping overtime . . . at one hundred hours. It is so easy to abuse the "yes" of a person who feels they cannot say "NO."

This is the depressing reality of what can happen when the body does not feel heard and we ignore its requests, because we exist in a culture that views our output as a measure of our value. If as a society we viewed our jobs as simply our jobs—roles we play—and not who we *are*, it would not cause an identity crisis to request a day off, or to state our need for rest. We might be more willing to walk away from toxic relationships, work environments, and situations. Our value should not be measured by the number of hours we spend playing a role or how well we play it. By slowing down and realizing that our "role" and our "true self" are separate, we create a gap between the role we play and the person we are. The secret to liberating ourselves lies in creating that gap. In finding meaning in our lives, in the areas that have nothing to do with our output, but in rest, in joy, in being.

Right now, we overvalue tangible, measurable assets produced from working and undervalue unquantifiable assets such as love, awe, joy, and rest that come from *being*. The latter traits are typically seen as "feminine" and therefore "weak." These are seen as less important because they can't be added to the quarterly spreadsheet or displayed on social media. They can only be felt. It is no wonder the planet is being destroyed—our obsession with overproduction is running it into the ground. If we can't measure something's growth in numbers, we don't want to know about it! We mostly prioritize what we can *see*—and discard the value obtained from that which we cannot see, such as love, contentment, joy, silence, stillness. It makes you question what our definition of success is, if we have no time to enjoy it.

"How we spend our days is, of course, how we spend our lives."
—Annie Dillard

Working hard is not itself a toxic, life-shortening activity. Self-discipline is one of the most rewarding skills you will ever acquire when it comes to making and sticking to decisions that are good for you. It is self-discipline that is going to help you fall back in love with your life, as you choose what's best for you, over what's comfortable. It is self-discipline that allowed me to finish writing this book!

But under a patriarchal society that has suppressed feminine energy in all humans, too many of us have internalized the belief that it is weak to slow down, show emotion, that our playful side is something to be embarrassed by. The idea that we shouldn't rest, slow down, and play is a hangover from the industrial revolution, to normalize the discontent that people felt working horrendous hours, and it is still alive today. We need to find joy in the mundane because for the most part, that is what we spend 90 percent of our lives doing. If we wait for our lives to begin on the weekends, or really start relaxing when we're retired, we will get to the end of our lives realizing that those sixty or seventy years we spent suffering in the hope of one day resting, *was* our life. Every single day we wake up is a day of our life. Your life belongs to you, with you, right now.

If you're feeling overwhelmed, and you're in that place of exhaustion right now, I am going to ask you to cancel something. I'm going to ask you to reschedule something. Look at your calendar, all of the events or favors you've tried to cram in because you feel pressure to give your days to others. *Move something*. If there's nothing to move, what can you cancel for yourself? Can you get an early night and put your phone in the other room? What can you do right now to claim back a sliver of your freedom? I want you to say "NO" to something and feel the space and the energy it gives you to remind yourself—one minute at a time, one canceled plan at a time—that your life belongs to you.

BEING SILLY IS THE ANTIDOTE TO BURNOUT

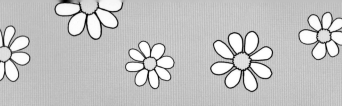
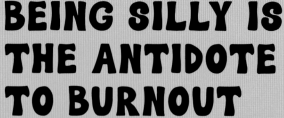

As a result of those years spent living in fear and chasing perfection—producing, perfecting, striving, goal-setting, *working, working, working*—I burnt out. I had left no room for the playful, sensitive, and spontaneous side of me to come out—the parts of me that were soft, silly, intuitive, playful—all things which are unvalued by capitalist society as weak, feminine traits that "prevent you from getting work done." And I too had started to believe they were inferior within myself. Femininity is something we have collectively suppressed for years, not just in men, but also in women. It is very tempting to ostracize those parts of ourselves, to abandon playfulness in order to be taken "seriously" by others.

I appear to be free-spirited, wild, alive—but I am *also* a massive control freak, riddled with perfectionism who's afraid of slowing down! My ability to be carefree is not innate, but a skill I have had to intentionally create over time, losing it, regaining it, losing it, forgetting it—it's a muscle that needs to be fucking strengthened! "Letting go" and "not giving a fuck" did not come easily to me. It took an active and conscious effort!

What other people see of my carefree self-expression is the *fruit* of the teamwork between both my playful inner-child *and* the structured perfectionist. You might not see the disciplined side of me, because most of it happens behind closed doors: when I'm working at my desk, getting myself out of bed early and working on deadlines, all to ensure the altar for my creativity is being prepared for the playful magic and expression to come out of me. The perfectionist in me prepares the altar, the playful child in me performs the magic on it. It actually requires discipline to be this playful! No magic in life can ever happen without the discipline for execution—and the execution without magic is dull. In the words of Eckhart Tolle, "Life is a dance between 'doing' and 'being.'"

Children's birthdays aren't beautiful without someone planning every detail. Family photo albums aren't compiled without someone intentionally taking pictures consistently throughout a child's life. The weekend away with your best friend, which bonded the two of you closer, couldn't have happened without booking the travel, accommodation, or setting the alarm early enough to catch the train. Every piece of magic we experience is usually planned or crafted by some organizing principle. Even if that organizing principle is simply the *decision* you make about where to place your attention, in any given moment. If a sunset lights up your path on a walk home, it is up to you to *choose* to marvel at it—and not pull out your phone to scroll through social media—for its beauty to chip away at your defense layer and allow the magic to touch you. There is always an organizing principle involved in creating and experiencing magical and joyful moments.

We are each in possession of these playful and structured energies, we have them within us, regardless of our gender. We require them to be working in balance within us to feel whole and life can feel a bit "off" when one is overpronounced in ourselves. Too much work and hustling can burn us out, and too much play can leave us craving structure and purpose. Life is full of responsibilities. School. Homework. Bills. Mortgages. Jobs. Roles. Profit. Loss. Deadlines. Organizing. Meetings. Chores. Calendars. These are all important and, for the most part, completely unavoidable. But any time I have lost myself in these roles and tasks, leaning too much on the striving part of myself, I lost connection to my joy. To that child inside me desperate to play and point out the funny, silly, beautiful things in life. She feels dismissed in the busyness, like an adult constantly saying, "Sorry darling, mommy's busy!" when a child asks to play. Life is about balancing these parts, without allowing one to govern all of us. It is when we are so heavily steered towards one or the other—too much play or too much hustle—that we suffer.

Globally, we are deeply out of balance, we are steered towards hustle. For a long time, we have feared the playful and feminine energy inside ourselves because we cannot understand it with our "thinking" mind. It rarely follows the laws of logic or reason but instead of intuition and flow, because that's what playfulness is—intuition. It is not something we "do," it is something we feel, something we know, a state of being. It follows instincts, it asks curious questions, it belongs to the realm of feeling that we cannot touch or see. Intuition is something women have incredible access to, which is why we have been taught not to trust it—we wouldn't be as easily controlled if we did.

It's not even three hundred years since the last woman was accused of witchcraft in the UK and burned at the stake. Condemned as a witch for cultivating and expressing her playful energy and using the powers of her intuition. What we cannot understand, we fear. When we fear something, we try to control it. We have distracted women so far from this source of power, by getting them to be afraid of it, mistrust it, giving all their attention to how they look instead. There has been a repression of feminine energy and an over-pronunciation of masculine energy globally, as a result of patriarchy and capitalism. We are all forced to adopt this structured, more masculine way of hustling in the world and this emotional repression is not only leading to our individual burnout but it is hurting our planet.

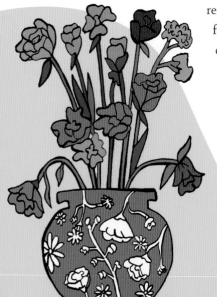

MOTHER EARTH

We need to look no further than the devastating effect that hyper-productivity is having on our planet, to see just how destructive this imbalance can be to our own bodies. The entire planet has been off-balance for too long. Under capitalist patriarchy, the intuitive, creative, and playful energy of human beings has been suppressed and shamed in favor of productivity, mass-production, and goal-oriented success at any cost—and just look at the state of Mother Earth. Look at what we're doing to her for our own endless craving to produce more, more, more! She is stressed, burnt out, she is being mined and fracked, the oceans are polluted and species are becoming endangered. She needs a break, she needs rest, she needs time to recover and heal.

When we are strictly goal-oriented and focusing on achieving an outcome, we are less likely to respect the journey of how we get there, and focus more on getting there as quickly as possible. We are less likely to make informed, sustainable, intentional choices and more likely to cut corners, burn ourselves out, harm ourselves or others, and try to achieve something by any means necessary. When we discard the importance of joy, of play and presence, we normalize the emphasis on working, of not enjoying life, of not finding joy in our roles and responsibilities. We normalize discontent. We forget that the journey is the most fulfilling part. We are our own little "earth." We too need a balance in both of these polarizing energies, of playing and working, of doing and being.

When we are severed from our playful energy for too long, we don't just lose our connection to ourselves, but we can also lose our connection to others. Just like the crabs in the bucket we discussed on page xx, we are coerced into developing individualistic tendencies to survive under capitalism in an "eat or be eaten" world, which contributes to us becoming more and more disconnected. Connection is what innately makes us human and it's what we are being cut off from.

REDISCOVER YOUR INTUITION

Our connection to intuition is so important in creating a life we desire, because it is the part of us that tells us what we *actually* want and need in the first place. We learn from the outside world to suppress this intuitive energy, perhaps through a partner who belittles us having other interests outside the relationship and views our creativity as a threat, teachers who diminish our curiosity and discourage us from asking questions, people we trusted who told us that we didn't see something . . . *even though we did*. The journey back to our intuition is through intentional connection. Quietening the mind into stillness, keeping those gaps open, putting the phone down for one minute, sitting on that mental bench, making our own decisions, and fine-tuning our connection to the sound of *ourselves* again. You will not discover something new, but rediscover what was always there. It's going to feel like coming home. It's going to feel delicious.

Whenever I am overruled by my perfectionist self—when I give myself no rest, no pause, no play, no joy, no fun, and fetishize my productivity—I receive a little nudge from my body, like a gentle whisper to slow down. This might show up in sleepiness. Or perhaps I become poorly. Or I get an ache in my body. Or I'm reactive and snap at someone. It took me so long to realize that this is bodily wisdom, not an obstacle to overcome, push down, or suppress or an inherent weakness. It is a calling from within to rest, adequately. Not by planting a screen in front of my face, but by sinking into "boredom" and seeing what visits me there. In my experience, these signals were the warning signs for burnout, and instead of listening to them, I tried to override them because the voice of my default self shamed me for being unproductive, called me a bad friend, bad boss, bad this, bad that. Often when this happens, many of us don't feel we have a choice. We go to work poorly. We join the Zoom meeting from our beds. We work until our bladders are crying out in pain. We go weeks without seeing friends. We don't eat properly because cooking and preparing fresh food takes "too much time," so we order something quick instead. Efficiency replaces care. But that voice doesn't belong to you, remember? It was planted into you. It is just a habit—and you can break it.

Unless you make an intentional effort to enjoy your life, that enjoyment will be side-lined, forgotten, until it's eventually deemed "unnecessary" for a

good life. Being silly, being playful, laughing, crying in awe, going for walks, reading books—doing anything that the perfectionist voice in me believes is a "waste of time"—has fucking healed me. It has resuscitated the part of me that felt dead inside, the part I thought had lost its spark, the joy I once had and started to mourn as a nostalgic and distant memory. Turns out, she never fucking left! She was waiting inside this whole time for me to slow down. Everything in our lives lights up when we engage the curiosity and the playfulness of that inner child. The inside-out glow of pursuing the things that bring us joy is unmatched.

During the pandemic when a lot of us stayed at home, businesses had shut, and cars were off the streets—Mother Earth slowly started to take back what was hers. Across the world, animals roamed the highways, birds returned to homes they hadn't visited for years, and the ocean's wildlife felt safe to return to normally tourist-riddled beaches, without our pollution and chaos. Nature literally healed when we all slowed down. I imagine the same for ourselves, the sense of playfulness and freedom we gain when we no longer have our actions driven by the fear of "being behind" in the rat race. Slowly, we reveal the parts of ourselves long hidden, parts that now feel safe to explore and venture into the world and our lives.

Turning this shit around starts with us. It starts with being silly.

AFFIRMATION: I am a silly woman who gets shit done.

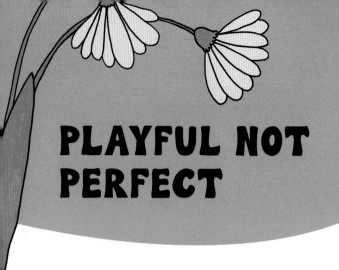

PLAYFUL NOT PERFECT

So what does playfulness look like in practice? For me, it starts with a cheeky little philosophy called: *playful not perfect*.

I want to be remembered as a woman who lived FULLY. Who laughed her ARSE off. Who was so joyful she was often misunderstood as high. Who loved her life so much that everything around her was touched by her joy. I want people to remember my energy. How I made them feel. How I helped them understand themselves. How I brought them delight. I want to be a woman so full of LIFE. But I cannot do any of this if I am still chasing perfection. If I am flat out exhausted from pleasing, or too busy obsessing over the way I look. None of us can. It's impossible.

How can people *feel* our presence and energy if we don't even fully occupy the space we take up in our own bodies? Lurking above like a witness to our own lives, instead of participating in them? To be a woman so full of life, we need to find ways to get back into our bodies. To get comfortable with making choices others may not understand.

Perfectionism and beauty standards stop us from taking action and jumping into our own lives. We miss the magic of life and spontaneity when we think we need to show up "perfectly" to everything. Perfectionism prevents playfulness! We stop trying new things. We skip the trips we want to go on. The events. Trying something new. All the stuff where living happens. Expansive and delicious living does not happen within the confines of our comfort zone. Most of it waits for permission, for enough "confidence" to find the courage to burst out of it. But in showing up imperfectly, precisely when we are "not ready," we can begin to transcend those limiting beliefs that have falsely told us we can only access life, experiences, beauty, joy, and living when we look good enough, or are "deserving enough." The way out of perfectionism is through taking action. That is how we break the feeling of being stuck in someone else's script. That is the only way. Getting back in touch with the playful, feminine energy inside ourselves, the one we experienced as a child or in brief intervals of creativity in our lives, lets us know on a cellular level that we are *already* enough. That we already possess the qualities that permit us to enter the world of living, dare I say it, *a delicious fucking life*. Taking action tells our brains we deserve to live that life *now*.

So fucking jump IN! Step-by-step, ignore the "perfect police" in your head and live your fucking life! When you make the goal of an activity to "have fun" instead of "achieving perfection," it will allow you the space to actually start living your life without fear. This could look like ignoring the voice in your head and going to an event, even though you don't have money to buy the new dress that your perfectionism is telling you that you NEED in order to attend. Why do you need to buy a new dress? Is this something that is actually written on the invitation? Or is it an additional layer of expectation your mind has placed on you? Is it actually a hangover from when your mom used to ask you to look "pretty" for family events as a child? Try to find where it has come from, so you can realize that it's not *you*. Consider what will actually happen if you just wear something from your existing wardrobe?

"Playful not perfect" means going on that date even though you are on your period or had a breakout (insert other excuse you use to stop doing brave things here). Working with your laptop from a café instead of at home and seeing what beautiful interactions happen as a result of you interacting with the world. Posting content online to connect with people even though you don't have the "right" equipment yet and just film from your bedroom on your phone. Going for a run in your comfy trackies despite the fact you don't have beautiful athleisure clothes and that you haven't run for over twenty seconds in your life.

YOU DON'T HAVE TO WAIT FOR **PERFECT**, YOU JUST HAVE TO FUCKING **BEGIN**.

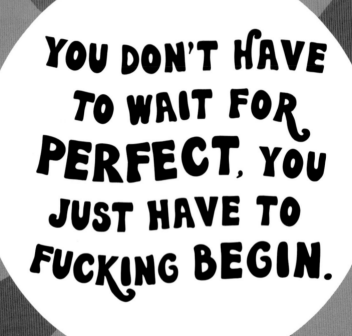

You don't have to wait to be perfect, you just have to fucking begin. The life you want is waiting for you. Often, the fear we have of not being "perfect" and of what others will say stops us from living the expansive lives we desire to live. Remember, this is your smallness training kicking in, convincing you that you're not ready, but you were *born* to bloom. To see *how* tall you can grow. To keep birthing new leaves and shoots any time someone tries to cut you down or undermine you. No one can undermine you if you do not let them. If you do not allow the seeds they sow to take root.

DRESSING UP IS SUPPOSED TO BE FUN

One of the areas of our lives that just might be the site of *most* perfectionism is getting dressed. Dressing up is supposed to feel good. It's supposed to be fun! Getting ready does not feel fun when we are imagining what everyone else will look like at the place we're going, or when we are doing it out of fear and using it as another opportunity to prove that we are enough. Femininity had felt for years like a performance to me, but only because it was something I thought I had to be "perfect" at. Releasing perfection from the way I dress and embracing playfulness has been one of the biggest changes for me in living a more carefree and delicious life.

As soon as I realized that I had this belief that femininity and "dressing up" was a way to receive love, attention, or to be perceived as "desirable," it made sense why the process of getting ready had stressed me out so much! Unknowingly, I was viewing it as a test of how "perfect" I could make myself look, instead of using it as a fun vehicle for authentic self-expression. When prettiness and femininity feel like obligations we need to perform, we can suffer greatly, trying to squeeze ourselves into these roles of who we think we "should" be and it smothers our joy, like an ill-fitting, itchy sweater. But instead of questioning if there's something wrong with the sweater, we start to think there's something "wrong" with ourselves for feeling uncomfortable in it, we believe there is something wrong with who *we* are. Maybe, you actually just need a new fucking sweater! If the way you express yourself no longer fits, try something else. Bin that itchy sweater of "femininity" and try on a new one, one that fits, that hugs you comfortably, that aligns with your soul, not your "role."

When getting dressed—if we feel like we want to scream, cry, throw our things around—we need to remind ourselves, patiently and out loud, that we do not need to be perfect. That we simply need to get dressed, decorate ourselves, and have fun. That we are getting dressed to go out to experience life, to meet new people, to open the portal to a new realm of possibilities. That is what leaving home is for! To EXPERIENCE. The dressing up part? *Who will you be today?* How will you communicate yourself with your clothes? That's just the fun part, the most EXCITING part.

HOW TO BECOME RIDICULOUSLY ATTRACTIVE

If you want to become attractive, become *authentic*. It might not be "pretty" and it might repulse some people. But that is the beauty of authenticity—it has a magnetic-like quality, where you repel the things that aren't meant for you but ALSO attract the things you align with into your orbit! People disliking you, whether you like it or not, is the magnetic nature of being authentic. It's nothing personal. It means it's *working*. It's the cost you pay for a life lived on your own terms. Authenticity is the single most time-efficient way of filtering out the things in your life that are not meant for you. Why delay the truth?

Magnets do not chase, they attract. A magnet does not change its qualities to find objects to connect with, it remains itself and *attracts* objects into its orbit. The same applies to us. When we stop reaching for things we think will make us look "desirable" and instead embrace the clothes and self-expression that delight us, we start *becoming* attractive. By choosing to do the shit we love—embodying so much more love, gratitude, and joy—we start to attract things and people who are compatible. There is nothing more attractive than a person who embodies these qualities. Think about it! Who would you rather spend time with? Someone who you can *feel* is pretending to be something they're not to win you over, or someone who radiates a love for their life so vibrantly, with or without your approval? My soul aches to be around authentic people. Even if I don't agree with them, there is something so infectious about the courage of a person who remains open to new perspectives, while refusing to dilute themselves.

I'M NOT HERE
TO LOOK PERFECT
I'M HERE TO
DECORATE MYSELF
AND HAVE FUN!

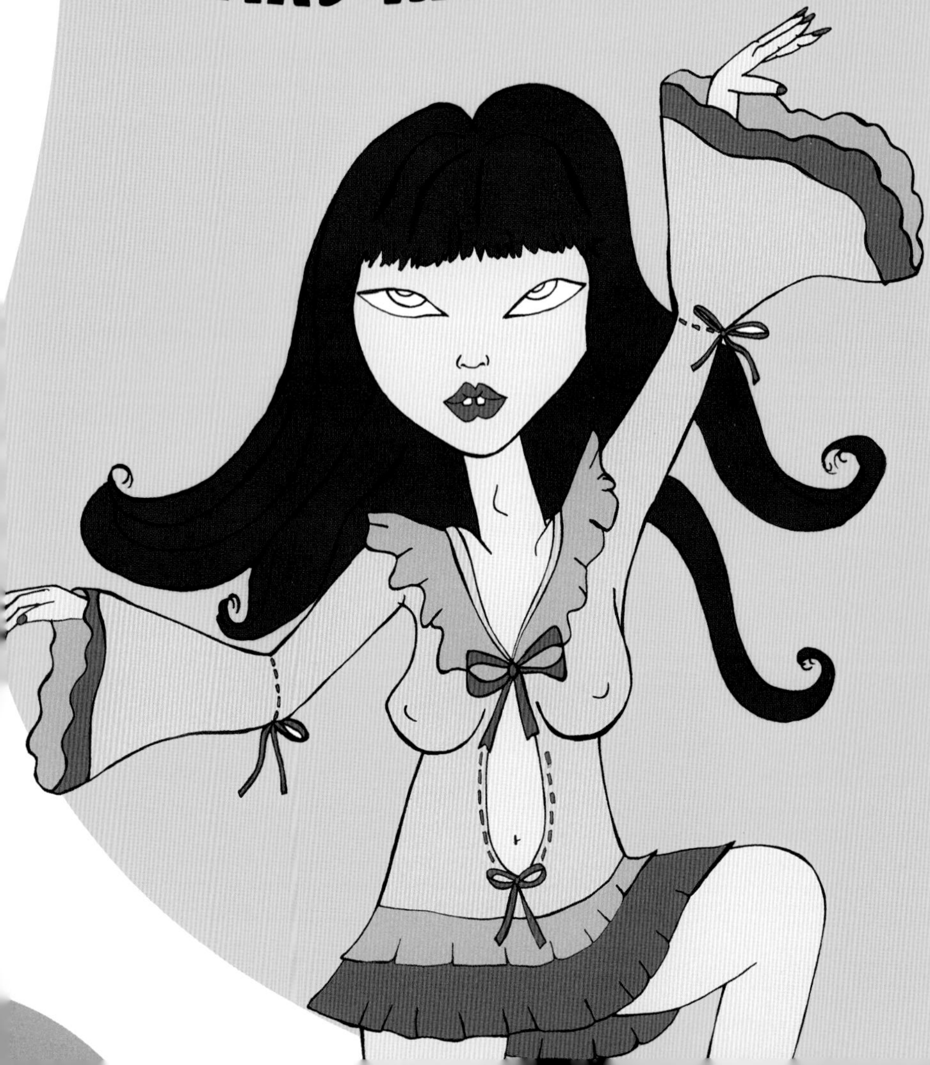

We glow differently when we FEEL good. I can sense even in photos of myself when I genuinely *felt* radiant and happy and when I was *trying* to look pretty and was actually filled with self-hatred. No matter how beautiful a picture is of me, no matter how wide my smile, if I know that I felt horrible while it was being taken I cannot enjoy the picture. It feels fraudulent. Our bodies are so good at detecting inauthenticity!

By choosing to be your authentic self, I'm not implying that you will receive the same attention, privileges, or desire from others that you did when you were conforming to "the norm." No matter how empowered you are in your authentic self-expression, the world will still barge in and treat you differently based on how you look. But the perks of choosing your authenticity over desirability are just different. Slowly, you care less about the approval of others and you get to actually FEEL good about yourself, independent of others' approval. Authenticity is a glow that cannot be purchased and will have people watching in awe thinking, *What's her secret?!*

When I stopped clinging to my need for "perfection" by choosing to show up whether I was ready or not, messily getting into action instead of theorizing in my head, the more I gravitated towards things that brought me joy, and strange, beautiful, and unexplainable coincidences started to occur in my life. In these moments it felt like life was winking at me, rewarding me for my courage.

We are going to go through why we cringe at authentic people later, but for now just know that you do not need to abandon yourself. You are so much more powerful (and sexier!) when you stay whole. Showing up imperfectly instead of waiting to be "ready" is what freedom looks like. It's not always going to be possible to make the brave choice. But taking small steps will bring us closer to the life of our fucking dreams.

We rarely stop to consider that people might love us *more* for not being perfect. What if the people we're trying to prove things to don't need us to prove anything? What if they still want us to come over last minute, even if we show up as we are? What if we radically make our own approval the center of our lives and make others' approval come second? What if authenticity makes us grow into the most attractive version of ourselves? What if we refuse to become the perfect hologram the world wants to see? What if this version of ourself is ENOUGH?

Playful not perfect.

Playful not perfect.

Playful not perfect.

AFFIRMATION: I am not here to be pretty. I am here to decorate myself and have *fun*.

My aim in this book is to guide you to learn the feeling, sound, texture of your own voice—not the voice of feminists, your partner, my voice, or your mom's voice—but *your* voice and how it feels within you. As we've discussed, it's not easy to learn which voice is ours and which voices we've inherited from fear or trauma. But with time, you will start to hear her. And she will become your guiding compass, your intuition, your wisdom. You will let her have the final say. You will learn to trust her as the judge of the council presiding over all those other voices you have within you.

You're going to discover her inside yourself so that you never look to others to outsource your power or your values again. No part of you will try to convince other people to see how *good* you really are, how *perfect*, how *pretty*, how *worthy*. Because you will know yourself and your self-perception will not be contingent on their approval.

You will uncover *your* true desires and build a life around *them*. Let's take a look at how we can fine-tune our connection to our intuition next.

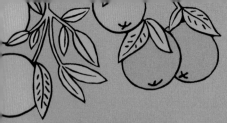

LIVING A DELICIOUS LIFE OF YOUR OWN DESIGN

Our desires are complex. Our desires are as complex *as fuck*!

How well do we really know ourselves and what does our "intuition" feel like? How much of who we are is *who we truthfully are* and how much of our personality is a response to trauma and social conditioning?

These questions are enough to send us into a head-fuck of an existential crisis. Especially when we consider the truth that who we "are" is largely a direct result of the conditioning of our environment. Most of our "personality" is a collection of habits we have built in response to our environment. For example, you might eat meat because it was normal in your family. You might drink alcohol because it's the way all of your friends socialize. Your friend group may even be based on who was in your school or in your area growing up. You never *consciously* chose these things, they have just formed as habits in reaction to the world you grew up in. But because we don't choose these sets of behaviors, when we change and grow without making any changes to our habits or lifestyle to reflect this inner shift, our lives can start to feel incongruent with who we are. Just like that ill-fitting sweater, life feels fucking ITCHY! As if something within us is squirming and writhing to be let out, expand, and bloom. Our true authentic selves can feel suffocated underneath all these layers of old habits and learned behaviors. Perhaps you realize you don't want to drink alcohol anymore, but still do it to fit in with your friends. Or maybe you have a desire to start dating women if you realize you like girls, a desire to leave your city, a desire to leave your job, to exercise, to make music, to write. When we change on the "inside" but continue to perform the old, habitual version of ourselves and fulfill the expectations that others have of us, we experience this friction in our lives.

For most of us, this manifests as an inner "itch." A new desire wants to emerge and bloom, but our mental resistance tries to push it down. But the desire doesn't go away, it just keeps nagging and starts to feel ignored and rejected. This is what creates deep shame. Often, it's too uncomfortable to examine this new desire because we have built an entire life around our old desires, and it means dismantling everything we have fucking built, to make room for something we're not even sure will "work out." We feel it's easier to just ignore it. We learn to rationalize the desire away as "insignificant" or a mere "fantasy" because we're afraid of shifting the world we have so perfectly built around us. The trouble is, the world we are in right now *isn't* perfect anymore. Otherwise, it would still feel right. Something needs to change and we know it.

The beautiful thing is that what makes us happy now, does not have to be the same thing that made us happy years ago, or the same thing that makes other people happy! The more we ignore our true desires, the longer we delay our freedom, the more life starts to take on the shape of our fears. Having different desires to the ones we had a year ago, or even yesterday, is totally fucking normal. We were never supposed to stay the same. It might FEEL like we signed a contract with all of the people in our lives to say, "I promise to always want the same things and be the same person" —but we didn't. Often, it may not even be the people *in* our lives that we're afraid will judge the new person that we want to blossom into, but people from our past, exes, old friends—the people no longer in our lives, but who live rent-free in our minds as judgmental critics, creating that inner council of voices. The guilt we feel for changing our minds and wanting something different can hold us in place, preventing us from growing. It can be scary to no longer want the things we used to, or relate to the things that other people want, but it's also a sign that we are finally listening to ourselves! This is exciting fucking stuff!

If we do not act on these signals, we can spend a lifetime chasing these things: acquiring new clothes, marriages, houses, kids, careers, or holidays, hoping the chasing will pay off once *we finally reach that next milestone!* Only to realize when we reach it, that it was someone else's idea of happiness. It was never our own.

It's often not the "big events" or the cars or the trips that make people happy, but the journey they take getting there. Take marriage, for example— getting married won't make you happy if the relationship you are *in* can't make you happy. We associate "single" with sadness and "marriage" with success. But there's a woman in the world right now who's single, alone, and GRATEFUL to have a life that revolves around her own needs. There's a woman who's married and wakes up every morning crying tears of misery, considering divorce, wishing she could be single. We should never mistake these emblems of life events as the means to happiness. Happiness isn't cultivated through achieving an "end" goal or one of these symbols, it's not an asset you can acquire. It's a way of being, one that we can cultivate and build through considered, intentional design, brick by brick. It's a feeling that comes from within, not something you acquire from without.

This is why generating a relationship with our intuition is key—it prevents us from striving for the things that make others happy and instead helps us to live intentionally, listening to what lights us up from within, and allowing *that* to be our compass. It could be being single with a child. It could be working part-time so you have *less* money, but *more* free time to do whatever the fuck you want. It could be cutting off all your hair to feel liberated from the task of brushing it every morning. Who the fuck knows?! Not me. Not feminism. Not this book. Not your mom. Not your mates. No one but you.

HOW TO LEARN WHAT LIGHTS YOU UP

For many of us, the idea of experiencing joy alone is unimaginable. I'm often asked, "How do you have so much bloody fun by yourself?" I have always been able to find a pocket of joy in my days, "even" when I'm alone (if I'm

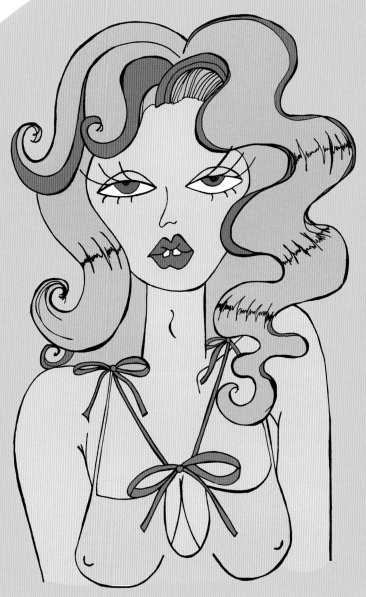

DESIGN A LIFE THAT IS DELICIOUSLY YOURS!

being honest, I often prefer it). Being a loner is the only way I have ever been able to figure out who the fuck I am! At first it may seem frightening to spend time alone, but that is how we learn if other people's company is something we are CHOOSING, or something we are using to fill the void within. Being open to having fun on our own and excavating our days for small pleasures ensures that our life is created consciously, not on default. Try to shift your perspective from thinking it's weird, pointless, or embarrassing to spend time alone, to viewing it as a fucking privilege, as the beginning of the process of courting *yourself*! Instead of pretending to like certain things to win over relationships with others, when you spend time alone you can engage in the things you ACTUALLY want to do and the things you love, to win over a relationship with yourself! The love of your life! The one that will never leave you! Get to know HER. What does she like? What is she about? How can you woo her?!

When we fill too much of our minds with the needs and desires of other people, outsourcing our intuition as we have discussed earlier, it can become hard to see clearly what we want for ourselves. We may run on other people's schedules, go to places our friends want to go to, dress in a way other people might, talk in the way others do, always presenting ourselves to "fit in." That's why time alone is crucial for us to find *our* center, what *we* actually consider fun and also what we *need*, away from the noise of others. We have been taught to believe that being alone is a sign of our unworthiness, or being a "loner," when in truth it's the only way to find yourself within your own skin. Being alone gives you a true understanding of how you are and who you are when no one is watching. When you are alone, your authentic self feels safe to rise to the surface. Very few people are willing to sit in this silence, which is why originality is so fucking rare—it requires uncomfortable periods of solitude to hear your own unique voice.

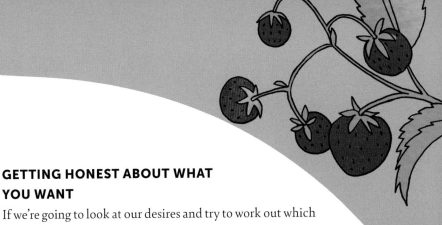

GETTING HONEST ABOUT WHAT YOU WANT

If we're going to look at our desires and try to work out which belong to us and which belong to other people, it's important to be brutally fucking honest about the things in our lives we do out of *obligation*—events, parties, hobbies, habits—whatever it is, make a note of it. It is the only way we're able to discern the difference between a "fuck yes" and a "fuck NO."

Of course, we all have roles and certain duties to perform that we can't escape—this is part of being a kind, responsible person. We all have to do things we don't want to do. But when it comes to our social life, or choosing our careers or partners or friends, there are so many things we forget that we can opt out from, in the fog of guilt and people-pleasing. We forget that we are the architects of our lives and that if we don't design them, they get fucking designed for us! We're going to have to be ready to make others uncomfortable with decisions we make about our own lives.

Learning to make choices about your life, *even if they make others uncomfortable*, is the key to freedom. We'll go deeper into how to set boundaries later in the book, but something that isn't spoken about enough is the discomfort we feel when we do the *right* thing for ourselves. We assume the "right" thing is supposed to "feel" good when it doesn't always, sometimes it feels fucking terrible! Feeling discomfort when we make the right choice can often trick us into thinking we made the wrong one. So we take the boundary back, we say, "It doesn't matter, you know what, it's not that big of a deal," and end up right back in the cycle of over-committing to crap we don't want to do. So, I want you to *expect* to feel like the worst person in the world when you make a decision based on what is right for you. Feel like a bitch, let the emotions pass, and hold the boundary. It is not an exaggeration when I say that your ability

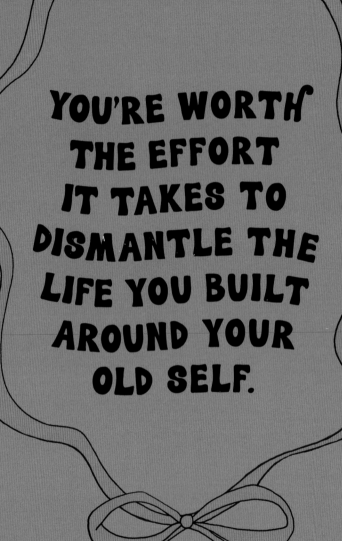

YOU'RE WORTH
THE EFFORT
IT TAKES TO
DISMANTLE THE
LIFE YOU BUILT
AROUND YOUR
OLD SELF.

to do this directly determines your ability to live a fulfilling life. Otherwise your life will always be shaped by protecting others' feelings.

If you're hearing this and wondering, *But Floss, I don't know what I want, that's the problem, that's why I keep pleasing others!*, do not worry. There is a secret hidden device within all of us that's going to tell you exactly what you want. You just need to learn how to tune-in to its frequency.

In the journey of discovering your desires so you can slowly inch closer to a life that is centered around your pleasure, your body is going to be your fucking BESTIE. She is going to show you and tell you *exactly* what feels good. You just need to slow down and listen to her. She can only be heard when you're not running around, numbing out, and ignoring her. She requires your presence and attention, just like a lover would. She is going to be the perfect companion in creating a life that you desire. Make a habit of simply observing the feelings in your body. When do you feel uncomfortable? When your heart clenches in conversation with a stranger because something feels "off" about them, do you ignore it or do you wrap it up and walk away? Who does your body feel most relaxed around, who provides such safety that it allows the child in you to come out and play and be silly? Does your heart pound before bed after you've been on your phone for hours? When is it relaxed? These bodily sensations are your teachers. This process of observation will help you obtain information about yourself and how you feel in certain situations, which is going to provide you the road map in creating a life of your design. Only then can you start to implement changes: the boundaries, the "Sorry I don't want to talk about my ex anymore, can we change the topic?", the "I'm busy tonight, can we do next week?", the "No I really can't get it done by the end of the day, it just won't be good enough." All of these assertions will help you create a life you enjoy, instead of one

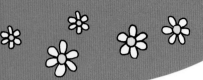

THE GIFT OF FEAR

Take note of the decisions you make out of fear. Like letting someone come over after a date even though you didn't really want them to. Take note of the decisions you made from joy, the ones when your body was screaming "fuck YES." Ask yourself the question, "Does this *sound* good to me, or does it *feel* good to me?"

Before our minds burst in and try to rationalize and intellectualize something, we feel it deep in the body. For me it's in my chest. My heart expands or it contracts, shutting down or opening up. It could happen around a certain person, when someone says something, a weird interaction on a night out, or a friend who somehow leaves me feeling confused about whether they just insulted or complimented me. That "gut" sensation we feel in the body is just information, but it becomes *wisdom* when we finally have the courage to act on it. If we keep a note—mental or physical—about our "gut feelings" and when our energy levels are high or low, we start to notice a pattern. Do we even feel good after gossiping? Are the hangovers worth the shit night out anymore? We can start to notice where the people-pleaser in us ignored that ping of danger or discomfort, in pursuit of pleasing others.

Our intuition is our inner compass that, once we learn to use it, will allow us to feel safer because we trust it to guide us. Women are socialized to be nice and kind at all costs, even when we are in danger, sometimes *especially* when we're in danger. This desire to be seen as "nice" muddies the waters of our intuition as we often dismiss our own instincts because we don't want to be seen as a *bitch*. In his book *The Gift of Fear*, Gavin De Becker shares stories of women who have experienced violent attacks by men. His aim is to prevent them from reoccurring by showing women how to listen to their bodies. Let me be clear: women are attacked because men decide to attack them. It is never a woman's fault if she is attacked, regardless of how in tune or not she is with her inner compass. But I urge you still to not disregard your intuition. In De Becker's interviews with victims, he asks if they saw a sign of the attack coming. All of the women initially offer some variation of the following response: "No, he was so nice! He offered to help with my groceries." But after a moment, they usually pause before adding something along the lines of, "You know what, now I think about it, something *was* off about him. My heart started pounding and I felt nauseous for no reason when he looked at me, but then I felt bad for judging him so I accepted his help and let him carry my groceries." All of these women received a signal from their bodies of danger but because of the culturally ingrained training to be "nice," it was suppressed by their minds. This intuition we have of something being "off" —whether it's physical danger or something as small as suspecting a friend doesn't have your best interests at heart—is our bodies' clever mechanism of picking up on inconsistencies and processing tiny fragments of information and behavior that our conscious minds don't have room for, or don't want to process. All of that information results in the bodily sensation we know as a "gut feeling."

For example, one woman interviewed by De Becker said that she later realized the reason she must have felt "danger" in her body, even though her attacker "seemed nice," was because she closed the door to her apartment building when she entered and when he came up behind her to offer help with groceries, the door hadn't made a noise. So he had already been inside the building, potentially for hours, *waiting* for her to come home. She didn't know this consciously—the absence of the noise was too small a detail to notice—but her body detected an inconsistency and alerted her to it immediately. The biggest take away from Gavin De Becker's book is this: as soon as your body feels in danger, honor it.

We can even feel guilty for changing our minds, betraying our desires so as not to inconvenience others. I have been on my way to a hookup before, knowing that I didn't

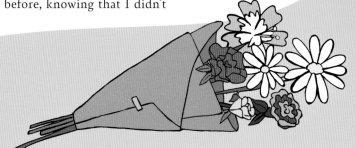

want to go, but feeling so paralysed by the guilt of "changing my mind" that I went anyway. It feels bizarre to say this out loud, to write this down, but guilt and fear drives so many of our lives. We experience so much guilt from changing our minds that we become very good at disappointing *ourselves* to spare the feelings of other people. Even if all we do is accept the cold dish of food at a restaurant to not "upset" the waiter, or smile at the hairdresser when we want to scream because we hate our haircut! All of these choices to *not* speak up and voice our desires compound. When we are frozen by guilt in this way, we forget that we can say "NO." But we can *always* change our minds, even when we think it's "too late." Stop placing the feelings of others above your own comfort.

Honor the true version of yourself by making the decision from this day forwards to leave as soon as the vibe feels off, leave as *soon* as you feel uncomfortable, leave as soon as you want. You can also honor your intuition by acting on your DESIRES! Acting on the things you know in your gut feel right for you, even when they don't align with the life you've created or the vision others have of you. Pivoting your career when it makes sense to you but doesn't make sense to others. Moving to a new city for a job that excites you even if it feels "risky." The more you learn to listen to your intuition, the less it feels like taking a "risk," it starts to feel like divine fucking guidance! You start to trust yourself a little bit more each time and life just gets fucking easier because there's no more debating in your head.

USING OUR DESIRES TO SHAPE OUR LIVES

Instead of morphing and contorting ourselves to fit into a life that *looks* good to others, but ultimately doesn't *feel* good to live, we can start by honoring those intuitive hunches—regardless of what people think. By listening to our bodies we can prioritize how our lives FEEL over how they

LOOK. Although it might "look" good to get a corporate job, and help you receive lots of praise from your parents, you won't FEEL good about it if you always wanted to be an artist. In order to discern what "looks good" from what "feels good" we need to consider whether the excitement comes from external approval or from *within us.* If we cannot stick to a decision without the external approval or praise of others, we are doing it because it looks good. Not because it feels good. This is a decision made from pleasing and it will pull us out of alignment. A decision that FEELS good is made whether people approve or not. Sometimes our desires will align with what others want for us and that's one hell of a bonus. But their approval cannot be used as the fucking compass! The compass for our choices has to come from within.

I use the phrase, "If it's not a fuck yes it's a no" often as it guides me to make only decisions that feel true as FUCK and aligned with the woman I want to be and become. Our desires change all the time and the steps we take towards creating a life that reflects them as they evolve are EXCITING! Learning what we like, who we like, and when the hell we like it creates a layer of bullet-proof protection from succumbing to bullshit. By this, I mean preventing other people's desires, insecurities, and motives from interfering with that gut instinct. When our connection to our intuition becomes strong, other people are less able to disrupt it. When we get clear on what we want and how desire or discomfort feels in our bodies, people can no longer *tell us* what we want. Our desires can no longer be dictated to us, they come *from within us.* We lean into the practice of being a curator of our own experience as opposed to a bystander, and this is exactly what empowers us to feel more confident in our ability to say "NO." No longer the woman waiting to be chosen, but the woman that fucking *chooses.* And THAT is how you deserve to live for the rest of your life.

DESIGNING YOUR LIFE

How do you keep learning about what is good for you? How do you sift through cultural messaging to learn the texture of your intuition? Just keep living. Experimenting. Fucking up. Learning. Making better choices. Being playful, not perfect. And if you feel that bodily "gut instinct" in the face of danger, honor it instantly and leave.

Now it's up to you to experiment—HOW EXCITING! How do you want your life to taste? Experiment by spending five minutes writing down the perfect morning routine for you, or the perfect week. What would this include? No screen time, a walk, exposure to morning light, perhaps waking up fifteen minutes earlier to have quiet in the house before people wake up? Reading? Do you want to create a bedtime for yourself? If you could snap your fingers and change your life, what would it look, taste, and feel like? Note down the times when you feel the most *alive*—not the most desired, not the most liked, not the most needed, not the most praised, but the most alive in your body—and you will find little clues in everyday life about what is meant for you. Through this experimentation phase you can see how different your energy levels are on the different days of the week. It's about gathering some personal data to help you better understand yourself. This is how you prepare the altar and the banquet for more JOY to be invited into your life. If you notice that you feel happiest and have more energy on the days you don't check social media in the morning, stick with it for a while! Watch the compounding effect that this has on your life. Watch how joy feels as she can visit you more frequently now that you have made your life into a magical altar for her to come to! How do you like your coffee? Your conversation? Your orgasms? Your time? How do you like to dress and when does that change? Do you prefer to stay in or go out?

You get to make choices for your life that people don't understand. It is not their life to live. You are not obligated to play a role that suits the way they see you in the world. Go off-script. Intentionally do the things you want that you're afraid will "surprise" the people in your life. Show them, don't tell them, that they can never expect a "certain" version of you. Break the mould. Do it. Liberate yourself.

As you experiment, consider some of these questions along the way:

- Who is it that you're afraid of disappointing by choosing yourself?
- Do you feel guilt for changing your mind? What happens if you push through that guilt and allow yourself to make a choice that people don't understand?
- Whose voice is it that tells you that you aren't good enough for happiness, to smile, to laugh, to not give a shit about how you appear?
- Who is it that you're afraid won't support you? Or who will be envious if you get the fuck out of your own way and live the life you want?
- Can you mentally tell them to fuck off?

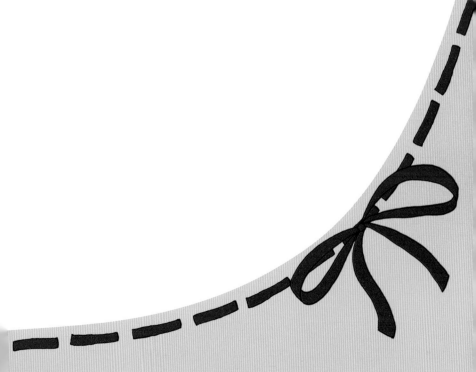

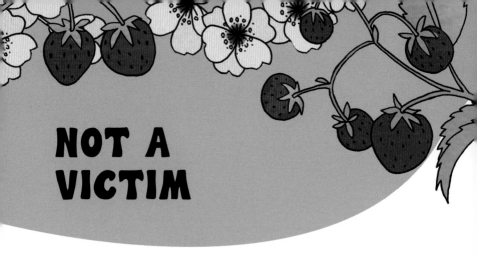

NOT A VICTIM

You are going to become more of an active participant in the decision-making in your own life.

Living a delicious life requires making conscious choices for ourselves that feel right for us, regardless of how other people feel about them. The trouble is, it's so fucking hard to access what we "really want" or how we "really feel" because of all of those voices blocking the path to our intuition. I'll never forget the anecdote that Glennon Doyle relates in her book *Untamed* about teaching a group of students and asking if they wanted sandwiches. The boys in the group, without hesitation, shot their hands up. The girls, however, all looked around at each other to decide if they were hungry, before collectively answering, "no." She remarks in dismay that the boys looked inside themselves for the answer, while the girls looked *out*. Just think about how many of those girls were hungry, but suppressed their appetite so they wouldn't feel like the "odd one out." We siphon power out of ourselves every single time we delegate the decisions of our lives to others and it starts so fucking young.

In adulthood this sounds like:

- "Sure, whatever you want."
- "Yeah, sure, that's fine!"
- "What do you think?"
- "I don't know, you choose."
- "I really want to do this. Do *you* think I should do this?"

If we constantly allow others to decide, we place ourselves in the passenger seat while our life gets designed for us and we can feel helpless. Some of the toughest pills for me to swallow when I was at my lowest, were that the world had the audacity to keep SPINNING when I was depressed (how dare it) and that no one was coming to save me. Staring at the ceiling light from my bed, feeling like my bones weighed ten tonnes, knowing that the only way out was through it, *fucking sucked*. Even when you've been through all kinds of fucked-up shit in life, the truth is the same: every, single, fucking, time—*no one is coming to save you*. Is that fair? No, of course not. But we cannot rely on life being "fair" to us for us to enjoy it. It sounds brutal, I know. It is. But the sooner we acknowledge that life owes us nothing, the quicker we are able to start changing our lives, right now. Even in that pit of depression, the only person who can get you to stand up and brush your teeth is yourself. Even though most of what happens in life is out of our control, we *can* control how we respond to it. We are not victims.

MAKING A MOVE ON YOUR OWN LIFE!

We can start to believe in our core that we are capable of changing our lives by transforming how we *see ourselves*. It is not enough to think differently, we need to take small ACTIONS that intentionally *oppose* the victim mindset of waiting for someone to save us. When we change how we view ourselves, we build the confidence required to believe we can design our lives. Even if the only thing we can muster the energy for is to open the window next to the bed to get some fresh air and hear the birds. It tells our brain: *I am not a victim. I deserve to hear the birds. I deserve to feel refreshed. I still love you even though you can't get out of bed!* This does not mean an avoidance of our pain or our circumstance, but an acknowledgment of our responsibility to get out of it. It is a gentle but defiant "FUCK YOU" to the depression, the ex, the abuser, or the fears in our heads. For me, that first step was simply choosing not to die. Then it was choosing to get dressed. Then it was choosing to go for a walk. Then it was choosing to Google "therapist near me." It starts with one step at a time. In every single situation.

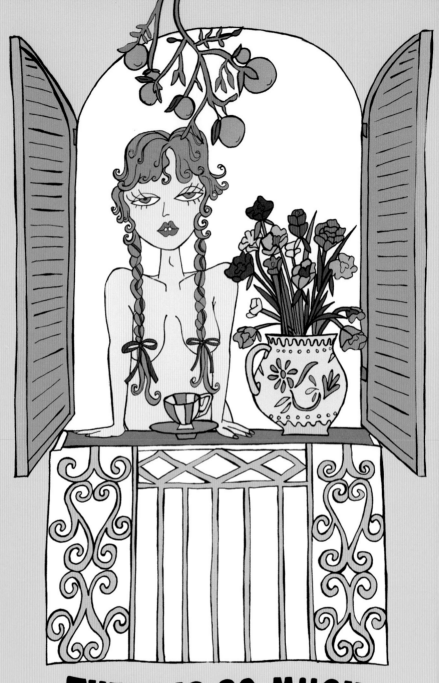

THERE IS SO MUCH
TO LIVE FOR!

The more we step into our own lives as active participants instead of passive voyeurs, the more we gain confidence in our ability to create our desired experience of life, the less we feel like victims. Taking action is the antidote to our feelings of powerlessness as it reminds us that we do have some level of control over our lives or, at the very least, control over how we respond to the events that unfold.

Albert Bandura is the most prominent researcher in human "agency," how much we feel we are capable of influencing our lives. Bandura says that people with high agency are "*producers* of their life circumstances and not just the products of them." Most of us, until we have a moment of reckoning which disrupts our world view, fall into the latter category. We are products of our environments and forget that we can also participate in the creation of our experience. We allow our environment to dictate the "ceiling" of our thinking and what we believe is possible for us. We assume this ceiling is the limit and do not consider that there is an entire expansive universe of possibility lying beyond it.

There are small ways we can reinforce our sense of agency. Like ordering something off the menu without consulting the other person at dinner, carrying a pen with you to write your ideas down when inspiration strikes, planning your outfit without asking for everyone's opinion, going for a walk instead of scrolling for another hour online, riding a bike if you've never tried it, trying new food, taking a different route home. These things sound small, but I can assure you they're not frivolous. These actions are the building blocks for developing agency, which will eventually build the confidence and trust in ourselves to know that we have the POWER to create our reality, through the concrete proof of our own actions. Agency is the antidote to helplessness. It is the antidote to the victim mindset. We're essentially building a reputation with ourselves so that in our darkest moments, something inside us reminds us, *We have done scary things before, remember? Let's fucking go.*

Often when we execute these little acts of courage, it is not the act itself that brings us an overwhelming sensation of joy and euphoria, but the agency and self-esteem we derive from making a conscious and intentional choice to change our environment without anyone's guidance. Bandura calls these "mastery experiences," when we build confidence in ourselves and our abilities by successfully completing a challenging task.

For example, when I discovered how happy the color pink made me, I decided to infuse it into as many areas of my life as possible. Everything from the color of my hair, to requesting "the pinkest room possible" for hotel reservations. I started to give my life a direction of joy, instead of following whatever was presented to me. But it's not just "pink" that makes me feel confident. It's the feeling I get from knowing that I am *intentionally* creating my environment to delight me. These things can make us feel powerful because they remind us, in small ways, that we can overcome the paralyzed sense that we have no control. It reminds us that we deserve to live deliciously, even if all we can muster is the energy to open that window and let the fresh air in.

To create more agency, you can start by writing or repeating some affirmations. There are some examples below, have a go with them and write your own to reflect your specific struggles.

- I will choose what's right for me, independent of other people's opinions, because when I allow my life to be shaped by other people's desires, l feel resentful. Choosing myself saves my relationships.
- I will order my own food off the menu instead of asking what everyone else is having first, because it's important to check in with what my body actually wants and how hungry it is.
- I will make a decision that feels good to me even though no one in my life "understands" it, because I am building a relationship with my intuition and that requires acting on my hunches to learn how it feels.
- I will control my reactions to my negative thoughts, because I am the master of them.
- I will go for dinner by myself even though it feels frightening, because doing scary things will build the confidence required for the person I want to become and the life I want to live.

- I will honor my gut feelings about people, even if no one agrees with me, because I would rather be seen as "cold" than rope another energy vampire into my life because I wanted to be "nice" and "agreeable."
- I will make decisions for my life and tell people after, because even if it's the wrong choice, I am happy to learn that lesson for myself and use this information to make better decisions in the future.

And guess what? If you choose the "wrong" thing on the menu, or you decide on an outfit that doesn't go as you desired, it doesn't matter—because your life is not a fucking test! Making your own decisions is not about getting it right. It's just about making your own decisions! Experiencing failure is the price we must pay in life for getting answers and information about what we do and don't want. There are no shortcuts to this wisdom. We are not supposed to get everything right. That was never the goal. Women are not supposed to be right all the time, or perfect. Just human. Maybe you ignored a gut feeling before making the wrong choice. Great! That's more info! Now you know how that feels, and you can apply this knowledge next time. Each time we get fucking stronger and wiser as we learn through these experiments what not to do next time. We learn the texture of who we are.

If you're someone who has always "gone along" with everything to keep the peace, I want you to intentionally do something that you've always wanted to do, but have avoided because of the fear of other people saying, *"Ooooo, that's not like you!"* or *"Who do you think you are?"* I don't want you to avoid that shit. I want you to embrace that shit. Why? Because you are reminding them and yourself that you are your own person, independent of the fiction they have of you in their minds. You are reminding them (and yourself!) that you are not just a side character in their lives who plays a role they're comfortable with and sticks to the script. You are your own main character at the center of your own story, just as they are at the center of theirs. Do the things you know will cause this reaction.

To take it a step further, instead of being nervous, I want you to get EXCITED at the anticipation of people making remarks about the new you.

DO SOMETHING THAT MAKES THE PEOPLE IN YOUR LIFE SAY "THAT'S NOT LIKE YOU!"

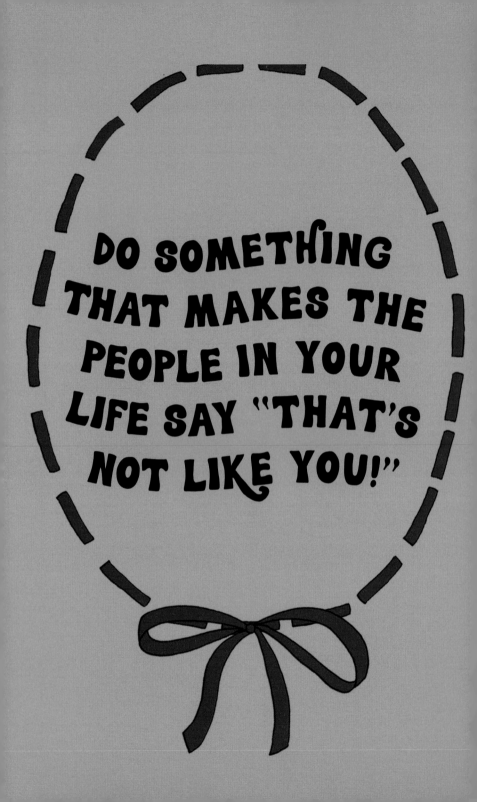

Get excited about people saying, *"That's not like you!"* You can reply back to them with an enthusiastic "Thank you, I'm actually trying really hard to not be like my old self!"

I encourage you to go off-script as often as fucking possible. Do something so different that it allows the fears of your critical inner voice to be deliciously contradicted, stunned into silence, as you show it with each disobedient action. Assert yourself to your inner critical voice . . . *I am not your victim.*

- I am not a victim to life.
- I am not a victim to my mind.
- I am not a victim to fear.
- I am not a victim to my habits.
- I am not a victim to the opinions of others.
- I am not a victim to the expectations of others.
- I am always the one holding the pen.
- I am always the one writing my own life.
- I am always the one who creates my experience of reality.
- I can always choose differently.

To achieve results you've never seen, you have to do things you've never done. You have to become someone you've never been. Say things you've never said. Read books you've never read. Position yourself in spaces you've never been. You have to make different choices. As obvious as it sounds, as much as we all "know" this already, it is a whole other thing to finally embody it. . . .

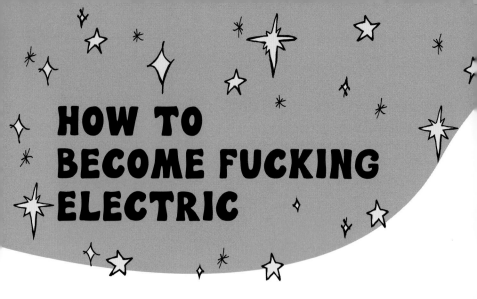

HOW TO BECOME FUCKING ELECTRIC

If you want to know how to become the most magnetic, electrifying version of yourself, you can start by asking yourself one simple question:

What habits do I have in my life that are not conducive to the person I want to become?

Why? Because for electricity to flow, there needs to be as little friction as possible. Asking yourself this question allows you to spot where there is friction in your life preventing that current from flowing, where you are being prevented from reaching your potential energy. Ask this question before you do something, anything. Suddenly everything becomes unbelievably clear. You can start to see the things you do every single day that this higher version of yourself would never do. *Would a woman who loves herself obsess over women online that make her feel like shit? No? So what would she do instead?* And then you do THAT! The aim of this question is not to change your life overnight, or to shame you, but to place a filter of awareness over your life and allow you to become more conscious of the small choices you make, and whether or not they align with the person you want to be. Often, the difference between the two is horrendously humbling.

BUILD A LIFE AROUND THE THINGS YOU LOVE

During my burnout, close to telling everyone in my life to "FUCK OFF" every single day due to my exhaustion, I realized that how I was living—

not prioritizing rest, sleep, eating, self-care_was not conducive to the woman I wanted to be. Not even close. The way I was living was not sustainable. So who *was* the woman I wanted to be? I had to literally write her down, listing all her qualities. I had experienced her in glimpses, on Sunday mornings when life felt slower and she had room to come up for air. I wanted to access that carefree version of myself with space to be generous and compassionate.

When we get very clear on the person we want to be, we can start to create a life and build habits around what we love, instead of on default settings. Love is a sustainable and motivating fuel to help us stick to positive changes. For example, on my list I noted that mornings are absolutely sacred to me. Yet when I wrote this, I was forced to see that I was not living in a way that prioritized them. I was going to sleep late, after hours of being on my phone, eating late, drinking alcohol, and waking up late—these were not conducive habits to gatekeeping my sacred mornings. Far more motivating than the idea that I would be "missing out" on a night at the pub or on hours of scrolling, the idea of a hangover-free life sounded pretty beautiful to me. This is what shifted me to change my habits. I realized I wasn't "missing out" at all, but "gaining more" of the things that fill me up—my mornings, sunrises, and increased levels of energy. This helped me build a loose routine geared towards my joy. When I started rising early, there was space around everything, there was a freedom that I felt was lacking in my life when I woke up and immediately shot into work mode. No longer did I feel the need to tell the people in my life to "FUCK OFF!" And I didn't buy anything to achieve this. It was like I unlocked a magical portal by simply changing what time I woke up and ensuring I prepared myself for this to happen, by changing those small habits.

If you want to be and feel fucking *electric*, you need to start by removing anything that is stopping that delicious current of electricity flowing through you. We all have things that bring us into a state of joy, clarity, and peace. We also have things that slow us down, deplete and drain our energy. If you want to be the most electric version of yourself, you must take small steps to reduce the friction in your life, so the current of energy can flow with ease through you. Just like a wire.

Energy leakage happens when we have poor boundaries, do things we don't want to do, and engage in old habits that no longer serve us. One of the most life-changing processes you can go through as a recovering people-pleaser is to patch up those leaks.

Examples of energy leakage and how you can plug them up:

- Gossiping that leaves you feeling grubby. Did it get taken too far? Did you say something you wish you hadn't? Next time you can try to change the subject.

- Too much screen time. The average global screen use is almost seven hours a day, which is almost nineteen years in an average lifetime. What a sobering realization. What might you be able to achieve, or feel, from simply putting your phone away?

- Having your phone out on the table. This is like a seductive portal of distraction! A black hole of attention! It feels like there's a third presence in the room. How much energy can you claim back by not having it on the table when working, on a date, or spending quality time with others?

- Crossing your own boundaries by committing to too much and going through life resenting the next event you signed up for. How about you cancel one thing this week?

- Ruminating without interrupting your thoughts. When your mind goes onto that autopilot setting, it can get chaotic up there. Try to take a deep breath every time you can feel the spiraling. Create more space in your brain. Go for a walk, do anything!

- Lack of preparation. If you know you find mornings stressful, can you prepare an outfit for yourself the night before, making it easier for you to get dressed in the morning?

- Negative friendships. Do you have a mate whose problems never seem to end and who constantly involves you in their emotional dramas? Can you take a step back? *What rules your mind controls your life.* If you're constantly absorbed by other people's problems, there will be no room for your own thoughts to create your life.

Remember, this is not about self-surveillance with the intent to punish yourself if you step out of line. The difference between self-surveillance and self-awareness is self-compassion.

The way I have best adapted my habits has been through asking myself about the life I want and getting detailed about what it would look like. Instead of being driven by fear, we can think about what we love and build a life around *that*.

BABY STEPS

Once we get really detailed about the person we want to become and we start to make changes towards becoming that person, we can get very excited, very quickly, and try to make a bunch of changes all at once. If you're one of the 91 percent of people who fail to stick to their New Year's resolutions, you have nothing to be ashamed of. It's obviously very fucking common! But if you want to be great and live a fulfilling life, you are just going to have to become uncommon and do the shit that a lot of people give up on. There's no shortcut to it. However, the reason most of us give up isn't due to a lack of discipline, but that we exhaust ourselves on the way to achieving our goals and they become too much to maintain. We dismiss the impact of small changes and try to climb the mountain before we've even stretched. Baby steps are the way to futureproof habit-breaking. Neuroscientists have found that we can only handle two new changes at a time, even if they're positive ones. We cannot move too fast, otherwise we'll burn out and turn "self-development" into another hustle.

James Clear, in his book *Atomic Habits*, says, "I have never seen someone consistently stick to positive habits in a negative environment." He also says that if we want to change, we should "make bad habits impossible" and "make good habits irresistible." How to make a bad habit impossible? Remove the distraction! It's one of the reasons I delete Instagram on my phone when I need to focus on work. Even seeing the app is enough to spike the dopamine in

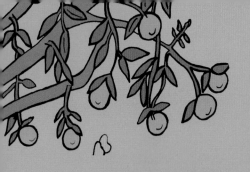

WHAT TINY HABITS ARE SLOWING YOU DOWN FROM REACHING YOUR POTENTIAL ENERGY?

my body and intrigue my curiosity to click on it and distract myself for hours on end. Why not eliminate temptation altogether? We need to make our environments as conducive as possible to support us, to stop the energy from leaking out and use it for what's important! Making your environment positive and designing it so that it is set up for success is the key to maintaining sustainable good habits. We are creatures of habit. Creatures of habit do what is familiar, not what is "good." So, we need to make that which is good familiar to us. It needs to be accessible. Exhausting our willpower every few weeks in short bursts isn't a sustainable solution and we are more likely to give up quicker. Not only do we become demotivated, but this solidifies our belief that we are someone who is incapable of making positive changes. Embodying the woman you want to become, tasting her in small doses—doesn't that sound more manageable?

HOW TO MAKE ADOPTING GOOD HABITS EASIER

James Clear calls it "temptation bundling," while other habit experts call it "habit stacking." We can use the high release of dopamine we experience in the anticipation of something we *want*, by pairing it with something we *need to do*. He suggests pairing the things we want to do with something we need to do, writing them out as instructions to ourselves. For example:

- *After I make my morning coffee, I will take a deep breath and stare out the window, observing everything outside for one minute of mental stillness.*
- *Every time I walk through a doorway into a new building or room, I will pause and take a deep breath. This will center me, bring me into my body, into the present moment, ensuring I have checked in with myself.*
- *After I brush my teeth, I will say five things I am grateful for and state an intention for the day (for example, "today I will use my phone less").*
- *Every time I unlock my phone, I will take three deep breaths. (You might just find you acted on an impulse and that you didn't want to pick it up in the first place.)*

These are some tips and examples that I use in my own life:

- When I feel the urge to complain, I replace it by saying something positive instead.

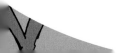

- I literally didn't have a habit of drinking water because there was no sink near me. As soon as I bought a pink, liter-sized water bottle, I began to drink two to three liters a day.
- I had got out of the habit of reading, telling myself I didn't have enough time. I knew the impact that reading had on my life and that books are beautiful portals we have into new worlds, so I tied the habit of reading into my morning walks, meaning I get in my steps and my reading time. A lot of people are shocked when they see me reading and walking, yet if I were holding a phone in my hand, no one would bat an eyelid.
- If you want to move your body more in the mornings, run in the direction of the coffee shop to motivate you to get moving. It's the only reason I get up and go in the morning—it's like a little treat waiting for me.

We can always be seduced back to bad habits—*You've had a long day, you deserve to spend time on social media before bed* or *I deserve a little fun, what's one night with my ex going to do to my growth?* It is next to impossible to stick to healthy habits in an environment that has been created to specifically seduce and target your desires. All of our bad habits are accessible to us if we do not change our environments. Let's not make it harder for ourselves!

HOW TO MAKE CHANGES TO YOUR ENVIRONMENT TO MAKE BAD HABITS IMPOSSIBLE

- Delete that person's phone number.
- Delete social media or dating apps from your phone.
- If you can't stop yourself watching TV until the early hours, hide the remote. Cancel the Netflix subscription.
- Turn the Wi-Fi router off to concentrate on your work.
- Leave your phone at home on your walk so you don't colonize that space for peace with the clutter of other people's lives on social media.
- Charge your phone overnight in a separate room so you don't scroll first thing in the morning. If you live in a studio flat, put it in a drawer. Make it as hard as possible to get to it.
- Buy an alarm clock or use anything but your phone alarm to wake you up. Otherwise, you may end up on Instagram before you know it.

- Delete the Instagram app before you go to bed to remove temptation.
- Don't have alcohol in the house if you want to quit drinking for a while.
- Put your yoga mat down ready for the next day as a visual reminder.
- Tell people you are not drinking before you meet them, so you have some accountability in place.
- Unfollow and mute the accounts that make you feel bad.
- Store a delicious thought for yourself in your mind which you can access when you start to feel anxious or need to soothe yourself.
- Get into the habit of listening to podcasts or reading books that provoke positive thinking in the morning.
- Block your access to being able to search for your ex.
- Write a list of things to do in a quiet moment around the house. If you have the impulse to slip into bad habits, start doing them!

Where are the holes in your life, where is energy being drained from you? *What things in your life are not conducive to the person you want to become?*

MORNING GLORY!

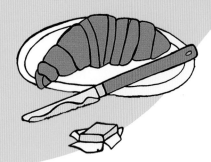

Early mornings are sacred to me. They are when I feel most "myself," outside of all life's responsibilities. Like a secret magical portal where it feels like time doesn't exist, where there is "space" around my coffee to savor it, "space" to get dressed without having to rush. The world is quiet, and streets feel like movie sets when all the actors and crew have gone home. The world feels, for a moment, deliciously mine. The thing is, I have to wake up early enough to fucking seize it. Otherwise, if I wake up too late, this magical slot of the day gets lost to life's responsibilities. Keeping my mornings free keeps me from resentment.

The second your feet hit the floor in the morning, are you someone else's *something*? You may be someone else's colleague as you reply to an email, someone else's partner as you ask them how they slept, or someone's house-mate when you ask to shower before them in the morning. We become so fluent in role-switching, we don't even see the energy it takes from us within half an hour of being awake. Our energy spills everywhere, before we've even poured it into ourselves. The world comes crashing in, leaving very little breathing space for the "you" behind these roles. We are instantly "on" and conscious of the people, places, and phone alerts that require our attention. The world rushes in and our desires rush out.

If we continue performing these roles every morning, over and over, without ever stopping to check in with ourselves first, we will never stop to see if our desires have changed or evolved. If our days begin as they always have done, we slip into the habit of playing the "role" of ourselves. We may find that we feel great irritation without being able to explain "why," without realizing it's because our lives have taken the shape of our old habits. The days are lived on autopilot! It's like we are sitting on life's train as it takes us wherever the driver decides—we forget we can check the map, get off at the next stop to change direction, and end up where *we* want to go.

This is how my life felt before I started waking up earlier. As soon as I awoke it was one thing after another, then before I knew it, it was time for bed. No room for contemplation or space to consider alternative ways of doing things. But the more aligned we are through checking in with ourselves, the more able we are to make decisions based on what we need, correcting the course as we go, with both "selves"—the role we play and the person performing the role—integrated. This is why I try to start the day with my feet firmly planted in who I am, so that I can course-correct through the rest of the day.

For me, a morning is a little "gap" between my authentic self and the "me" I present to the world. Without that gap, I can easily forget who I am. I can start to take the roles I play too seriously. In those early hours that I carve out for myself, I am left to sit in peace. After that, I feel less resentment for the things I have to do, because my cup is now full.

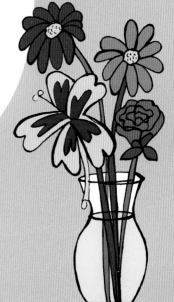

I'm not a morning person because I want to hustle, or be the girliest Girl Boss that ever girl bossed, or be the most productive version of myself I can possibly be—I am a morning person because I want to do "nothing." I do it because I yearn for and need unscheduled, delicious, do-whatever-the-hell-I-want time. I want to do "nothing" before 8 a.m. as it allows me to take this little slice of peace throughout my day. So I can be there and show up for the people I love and care for in the ways that they deserve.

Initially, you may feel guilty for filling your own cup first, but you have to trust in your generosity. That this pool of energy you generate for yourself will ripple out and impact everything in your life for the better. The people in my life didn't see that compassionate version of me for a while. Ironically, the running around I did for everyone else made me bitter. Martyrdom is one hell of a drug that we sell women to get them to place their attention, energy, and resources into everything and everyone but themselves. Refuse to participate. Refuse to dilute. Stay potent. Preserve your gaps. Trust that everyone, including yourself, will benefit.

SUNDAY MORNING IS A MINDSET

When do you normally feel the greatest sense of ease in your week? I feel it on a Sunday morning. Maybe an alarm doesn't have to be set and you're free to wake up when your body decides she has had adequate rest. Maybe you go for a morning walk, with more time to walk to the nicer bakery that has your favorite pastry. Or call your mom. Or watch that movie on your list. Sunday is often our only unscheduled day. If we are lucky, it's the time in the week when most of our minds come up for air and for a little while are free to wander, to dream, to think about the ways we want our lives to change. Some businesses shut on a Sunday, people seem friendlier—they are a little more contemplative and walking slower. Walking their dog. Less reactive to someone bumping into them. Coming back from a one-night stand. Hungover groups of friends filling cafés for the greasiest fry-ups. Maybe you go to church. On these collective days of rest, we tend to all lean into a temporary mental relief from the burden of our roles and responsibilities, soon to greet us again on Monday morning. This little pocket of the week was carved out for us specifically to do nothing. To appreciate what we have. To dream. To melt into the moment.

Sunday mornings have in many ways been a lesson to me: no matter what is going on in my life, the choice to see the beauty in the world is always there. To notice the things I mentioned about people_how they are, how they eat, how they rest on Sundays. The mundane beauty of everyday life was *always* there, it was just buried underneath the negative thoughts, the pain and the stories and the stress caused by the working week. Sundays always remind me that I need to make the seeking of beauty intentional, not an afterthought, not something left up to my environment or dictated to me by the schedule of my week.

This led me to wonder whether we could allow ourselves a "Sunday morning" on any morning, without the outside world permitting us. Could Sunday mornings in fact become a state of mind? Even if only for a few seconds? A state of mind in which we teach ourselves to believe that we have time, that we can afford to be slow, that there is no rush? Could we try to feel this way on Monday morning with a busy workweek ahead, or on a Thursday when we have dinner to cook, chores to complete, people to help? *Could I convince my anxiety that it's a Sunday morning whenever I want?*

If the external conditions that permit our minds to rest and exude gratitude on a Sunday allow us to be slower, then surely there is a way to achieve this the rest of the week? In fact, would moving about my life more slowly, more intentionally and consciously, actually improve my work performance during the week? I realized I had delegated relaxation and joy according to my weekly calendar. One day never felt fucking enough! There had to be a way I could trick myself into a Sunday morning state of mind. I decided to pause, carve out five minutes of my day to have coffee and not rush it. I considered whether if I woke up a little earlier I could find space for that slow, abundant, generous self every day. I wanted time in the morning to be filled with the things I didn't have time for during the day, the peace, the stillness. I didn't want to miss these little joys that were so crucial to my happiness. So that's why I decided to wake up earlier. This is how my mornings became sacred to me, when I decided to *make* them sacred. We are encouraged to rest when and only when we are told to rest. You may wake up at the same time as your partner, without even considering that you can get up earlier. Or that you can skip a late event. Did you know that you are allowed to experience joy and live your life whenever you want, not just on Sunday, not just when other people do? I didn't!

Living deliciously means finding our "Sunday mornings" in the everyday. There is a Sunday morning in your lunch break. There's a Sunday morning in your commute to work. Living deliciously is to claim rest and joy when we want it, so that we do not get to the end of our lives realizing that we were always chasing it in some unpromised, future moment_neglecting what was in front of us. It might be five minutes in the morning to ourselves, or two hours in the evening. I understand we all have different schedules, but I bet you can fit two minutes of stillness into your life. We can't afford to put joy last anymore. No one wants us to know that we're able to enjoy our time as we please, because if we start to find small, accessible paths to enjoyment we might realize so many of our consumer habits are pointless. We might realize that pointless striving is futile, boring, and leads to a perfect state of constant urgency where we make impulse purchases that leave us feeling more empty afterwards. That these purchases are just a distraction from what we were put on this earth to do: to enjoy our fucking lives, right now, in the present. Otherwise, we might blink and miss it all.

GOD. I WAS FUCKING MADE FOR THIS!

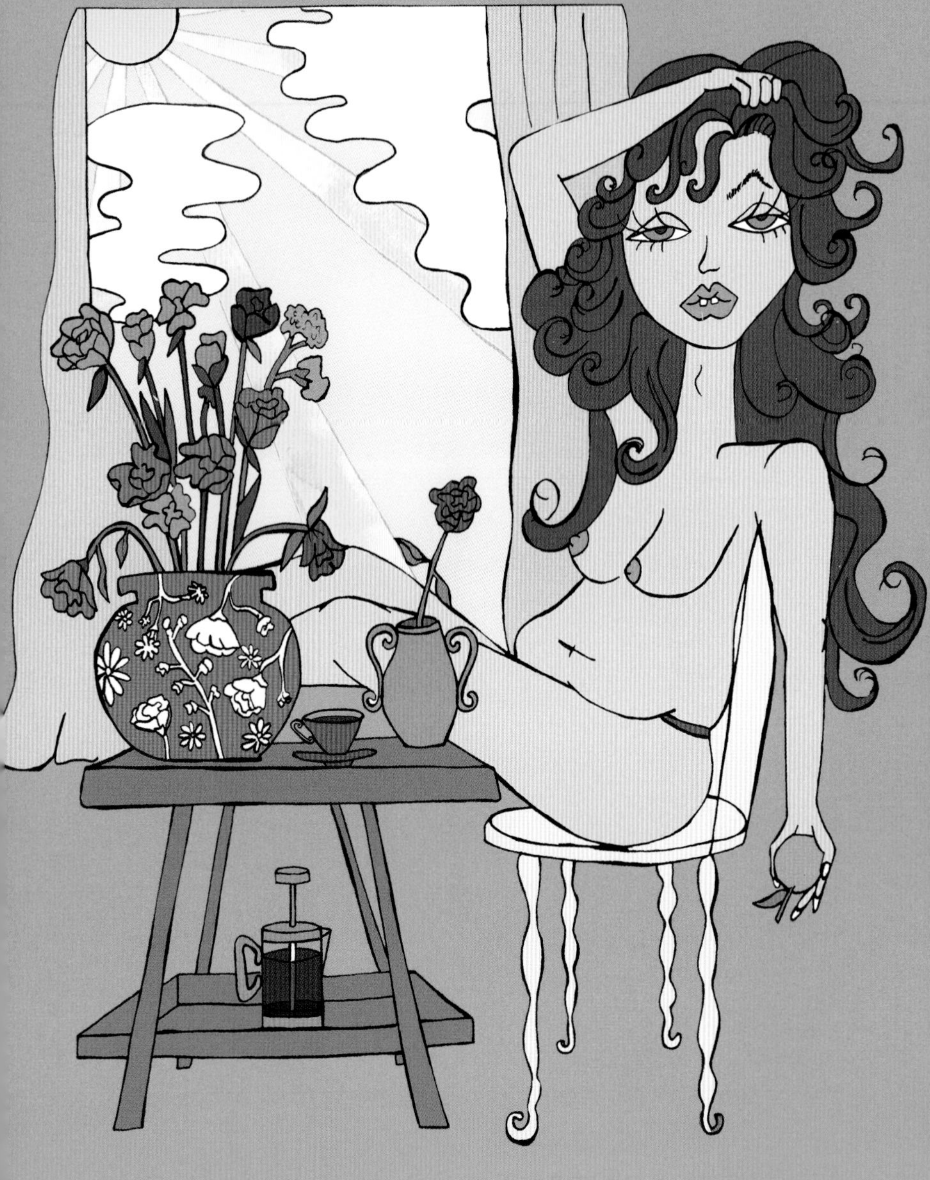

HOW TO EXPERIENCE SUNDAY MORNING BLISS EVERY DAY

- Before you drop something to help someone else, if it's not urgent, tell them you need five minutes. Or a day. Or tell them "not now." Often, we make other people's urgency our issue because we feel like a bad person for not immediately helping others. It isn't your problem, you can communicate that you need time. Delaying decisions on things people ask of me has restored so much power and agency into my life. Not everything is urgent, or needs to be done in a rush.
- Tell people you need a day or two to get back to them. For people-pleasers this is essential. We might need a bit longer to be able to check in with ourselves and see if we can really do something. But that doesn't mean we have to ghost the other person—we can text or call to let them know we need time to think.
- If your life is too busy for joy, too busy to stop and watch a sunset and feel the opening that it creates within you for love and connectedness to pour out, ask yourself what kind of a life have you created and what can you now, in this moment, dismantle in order to prioritize that connection to yourself?
- Cancel something. Schedule time in your dairy that says, "ME TIME." If someone asks if you're free that evening for drinks, guard it, say you're busy. For me, it meant canceling my subscription to streaming services temporarily to kick the habit of binge-watching a series before bed. It is impossible for me to just watch one episode. And if I can't do something in moderation, it's a habit that needs to be kicked. This then freed up my time to go to bed earlier, which meant I could wake up earlier and have two hours in the morning before any of my meetings to go for a walk!

Create that Sunday-morning feeling for yourself, every day. In small pockets. Your life does not begin in your sixties or seventies. It does not begin on Sunday. I know it may feel like it does, but is there something—anything—small that you can delight yourself with on the other days of the week to remind you that your life belongs to you? These days, the non-Sundays, they count too—they make up 85 percent of your life. Do you want to write that off? Can you find one thing in your day to bring you joy? Can you dismantle something in your life to create space for it? You don't just deserve peace or joy when the conditions around you ensure that nothing pesters you. You deserve it now. Don't disrespect your life like that. It's a gift. It is not unlimited. Your days are counting, so make them count.

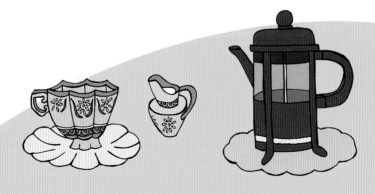

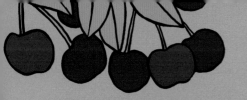

THE NECESSARY ART OF ROMANCING OURSELVES

Forget everything you've ever learned about romance. Creating more romance in your life does not require resources, money, or time. Just as you've identified your gaps to thread joy into your day, all that romance requires is your *creativity and intention*. It does not require you to do more, but to do what you already do *differently*. Like most things in life it is a skill, a way of *being* and a way of *seeing* which can be learned. Romancing yourself is at the core of creating a life from which you do not seek to be saved or rescued. *Why?* Because if you can create an absolute banquet out of your life, satiating your appetite for joy, delight, and romance, you are less likely to settle for the crumbs and scraps offered up to you by others. You need to learn to sweep yourself off your own fucking feet!

What would you like more of in your life? More sunsets? More space around your morning coffee? More laughter? More nature? More dancing? More joy? More creativity? To incorporate more of what you love into your life is a deeply romantic act. It is to treat yourself as a lover whose interests and joy are worth investing in, to make yourself feel special. A life forged from your design and intention is inherently romantic. At first, the idea of romanticizing the mundane moments in our lives can sound overwhelming, especially when we're *Women Living Exhaustedly!* You can't even find the motivation to strip and wash your bedsheets, and now this audacious woman (me) has the nerve to suggest you have the time to "romance yourself"? But this is precisely the point of making romance a sustainable habit, just like any other, so that it becomes so baked into our lives it becomes a way of being. Often, the reason we feel resistance to the idea of taking time for ourselves goes deeper than simply a lack of time—a lot of us also feel selfish. *How dare I take a moment of self-indulgent romance and luxury when there is so much to do, so much going on in the world?* A lot of us don't even know HOW to relax.

To many women, a single moment of joy or relaxation can induce such huge amounts of guilt and shame that it feels as though we have thrown everyone we love under the bus to take time for our silly, frivolous, and selfish little pleasures. This is no exaggeration. This is not hyperbolic! This is how it can feel. It is this guilt and discomfort we feel that controls and shames us back into the cage of pleasing, putting everyone first before ourselves. It's the thing that stops us asking for alone time. Stops us announcing we need five minutes to have our coffee. Women have said to me that they have wanted to give the flowers they bought for themselves to someone else, because they felt so guilty for buying them, not wanting them on the table for others to see. It is no surprise that we may feel rattled or even resentful at suggestions from others to take time out to rest, or feel a sharp bullet of hatred when we witness another woman appearing to be carefree, enjoying her life. In a world where taking time out from our roles is deemed selfish, an almost childlike voice inside us may want to lunge out and say, "Why HER? Why does SHE get to relax, it's not fair!" Relaxing and taking time out of our roles can feel as though we're betraying our family, friends, partner, or the entire feminist movement any time we have a moment of joy. Martyrdom runs deep. We find women on the brink of illness stumbling into work, apologizing for being poorly and for not being their normal spritely self. I fear as the years go on and we continue the good fight, we may miss the point of feminism entirely. We should be fighting for women to have ease in themselves, to be the gatekeepers of their limits. We should be fighting for women to enjoy their lives, to be their authentic selves, to explore what life can offer in the increasing freedom that was not afforded to our ancestors, while pushing the needle forwards for future generations. Getting proper rest and incorporating what we love into our lives helps us to be more compassionate and energized for others, with nervous systems ready to take on life's problems. It is odd that society admires those who appear physically exhausted and debilitated by their work ethic, despite usually being healthy and energetic, more than those who actually prioritize their rest and are able to contribute a hell of a lot more from this abundance! We need to flip the script. We need to see what the world would look like if we allowed ourselves to relax.

YOUR PLEASURE AT THE CENTER

To live deliciously is to ask ourselves, *How can I make this moment more beautiful? How can I enhance this experience?* This reminds us that we do not have to merely slog through everyday life, trawling from one thing to the next, but that a possibility to enjoy the journey, which consumes the majority of our lives, is always available. Making the moment more beautiful could be deciding to eat lunch outside on a sunny bench instead of in the office. It could be playing music while we cook, lighting a candle to start our day of work from home, taking the scenic route, leaving for work earlier to get our favorite coffee on the way. I like the moments of my life to be soundtracked with music, through earphones or on a speaker. I like flowers on my desk. I burn incense to fill the room with scent to invigorate me—I pack it when it I travel, along with a pink scarf to drape over a chair in the hotel room so that I notice a pop of my favorite color everywhere I go. It is these small pleasures that have always topped me up with a daily dose of joy. They sound trivial, but my god does life taste more delicious with them in it. These are the things that can enhance my experience of life, wherever I am.

Romancing ourselves and carving time out to do it is one of the most beautiful ways to access joy and amp up the sense of agency and control we feel over our lives. But that doesn't mean it won't feel completely, embar-

THE NECESSARY ART OF ROMANCING OURSELVES

rassingly fucking pointless at first. I sometimes find myself wearing pink ribbons in my hair or drinking coffee from my floral teacup and throwing my pink scarf over a hotel chair wondering, *Is all of this silly?* But no. It's not! Not if it brings me happiness! Not if it's going to energetically shift my mood, change the way I walk into rooms and interact with people that day. Remind yourself over and over that your happiness is generous and contagious. Remember? It's spilling out of you, always. You might find yourself thinking, *What's the point lighting a candle for dinner if it's just me? What's the point in booking a trip if I have no one to go with? Cleaning up? Dressing up?* With social media now such an integral part of our lives, a lot of us have bought into the idea that if something goes unwitnessed, it may as well not have happened. We forget that our own lives are sacred, worthy of having love poured into them for the sake of love itself—with or without receiving social praise. That's why these small things require a little bit of faith—the effects aren't tangible at first. We can't touch them, but we can feel them. It isn't just the "thing" we do that brings happiness. It's not about the flowers themselves. It's that when we look at the flowers, we know that WE created our environment to delight us *intentionally*. It's that wonderful hint of agency—the antithesis of feeling like a victim—that makes these small things feel so fucking good.

But, I don't want the practice of embracing romance and joy to become another exhausting performance of womanhood you feel you must carry out. It does not have to be pretty, it just has to delight you a little bit. You can take steps towards a life that delights you, whatever that means to *you* personally. Remember, my things won't be your things. My teacup and saucer with the birds chirping might be your flask of green tea on a hike at sunrise. Romancing yourself involves doing the things that make you feel good and doing them frequently, engaging with the most magnetic version of yourself as often as possible. Bathing in that frequency as often as you can. Becoming someone new, to get those results you've never seen before, in your life.

There's a wonderful saying: "You don't reap the crop the day you plant the seed." When you start to practice creating more joy in your life, think of it as a seed you've planted that you will have to keep watering, trusting it will grow and grow until it flowers. You have to be patient. You have to believe in the process of growth.

I know how fucking vibrantly I glow when I take care of myself, when I nourish my soul instead of starve her. When I go to bed early so that I can wake up feeling rested. Once we get a glimpse of that version of ourselves and we have tasted her, it becomes harder to justify going back. It normally takes a few weeks of consistently sticking to a new habit for us to start seeing measurable results, but one choice really can set our lives in a whole other direction: feeling excited to start the day because you prepared a cute tea set for yourself the night before, or have timed your alarm to ensure you catch the sunrise. These small things that generate excitement in our lives carry into our mood, our work, our relationships, our families, our creativity. What kind of work might you create from a place of enthusiasm instead of fear? Wouldn't it be great to find out? You may just feel that you're able to get out of bed without sulking. And isn't that alone worth *everything*? Isn't your life, this ONE fucking life, worth living with even a little bit more ease? This is the mere knock-on effect of feeling good, of centering pleasure in your life inch by inch. Your life is worth it.

ROMANCE IS CONTAGIOUS

Researchers have discovered that one of the pillars for cultivating self-esteem in our lives takes place through what are called "vicarious experiences." Which basically means believing something is possible for us by watching someone else achieving it. This is why women typically have lower self-esteem, since we do not get to see other women represented at the top of our careers or institutions, or women standing up for themselves. If we do not see people like us being treated with respect, we come to tolerate treatment at this level and assume that the things we want aren't possible for people like us. On the positive side, when we *do* see people like us thriving, we start to believe it's possible for us to have a similar journey. When we see a woman we know break up with her partner and flourish, we begin to believe we deserve better too, we see that it is possible to leave and fucking thrive! When we see a woman live by herself without a partner and become happier, we begin to realize, despite what our parents might say, that being single isn't a negative thing. When we see women perfectly fulfilled, relaxed, taking time for themselves, we believe we can do this too.

I once interviewed a therapist who said she starts every day with a bath, because "why wait until the end of the day to relax?" Another woman who blocks people on Instagram the second they say something she doesn't like on her page. It is through witnessing other women relax, set boundaries, and gatekeep their time that I have been able to model it and believe that it's possible for me. When we take the time to romance ourselves and prioritize our happiness, it allows us to gently influence other women in our lives—our daughters, the girls at work, our partners, the women who see us living an uncaged and delicious existence based around our own values.

We teach the people around us that romance doesn't have to be reserved for romantic partners. That we can be active participants in creating romance in our own lives. That we do not have to live our lives waiting for someone to come in and sweep us off our feet and save us. Imagine a world where girls grow up witnessing the lives of women who embody their own values, that live lives centering their own pleasure? Girls watching women at the center of their own fucking lives, would themselves grow into women who believe their values matter more than those of the society around them.

THE DECADENT AND NECESSARY ART OF SELF-ROMANCE

Romancing ourselves is not something we pick up when our self-esteem takes a hit. It should become a devotional practice and commitment we make to ourselves which reminds us that we always have the power to do something small to make our lives worth living.

A very capitalist idea of romance has been force-fed to us: red roses, Champagne, dinner at the swanky restaurant, a new outfit to get our date to fancy us. Yet we can do all of these things, go out with the right person, and *still* feel something is missing. Perhaps it's not that there is anything wrong with us or the person we're with, but that we're both engaging in an empty, shallow, one-size-fits-all version of romance that doesn't suit us. Just as the roles we habitually perform in our lives can exhaust us when they're ill-fitting and inauthentic, so too can an outdated version of being swept off our feet! It can leave us feeling hollow. The amount of pressure we culturally place on romantic love to fulfill our lives is also to blame. We think falling in love will be the solution to all our problems. But it isn't, and we are left feeling desperate when it doesn't fix us.

What I have come to learn is that romance is only truly effective when it is integrated and baked into our lives. When it is informed by what brings *us* joy, instead of what others collectively deem to be romantic. Choosing to walk on the sunny side of the street. Putting an album on to fill our home with delicious euphoric sounds. Sitting on the top of the bus with a fucking incredible playlist as it rains and watching the neon lights blur through the raindrops on the window. There is a refreshing aftertaste of agency and confidence from having created a moment all for ourselves, instead of buying "off-the-shelf" romance. This is why creating "gaps" in our lives is so important as they provide us with space to consider how to make the small moments even more delicious. Perhaps for you this looks like closing your laptop and taking yourself to sit and bask in the last hour of sunshine. Or buying yourself a pillow spray so when you come to bed later, it will feel so sacred to get a good night of sleep. What a luxury!

Creating romance in our lives makes us less susceptible to when people "use" romance to win over our affection. It makes it that much easier to walk away. If we are used to romance, if we *expect* romance because it is a habit—a way of being in the world and seeing beauty everywhere—other people's gestures cannot be used to sway or manipulate us. A romantic way of being also inspires and influences others to meet us at this level of treatment, without even asking or begging for it.

Have you ever dated someone who, after wining and dining you, was disappointed you wouldn't sleep with them and ghosted you immediately after? Or maybe you've seen a friend go through this? This person who wined and dined you was using romance to *get* something, using romance as a means to an end. When they didn't get the outcome they desired, the romance was no longer of use. Romance, true romance, is about the intention we put into something and enjoying the act of giving *itself*. Even if it's only leaving a handwritten thank-you letter to a member of staff who helped you, paying for your friend's favorite snack, or texting someone "good luck" before they have something important coming up. It's about the thought you have put into something for someone you love, including yourself, to care for them and make them feel special. Do something nice and don't fucking tell anyone about it. Try it!

We live in a society that praises the visible assets we can measure, while ignoring the invisible assets of love and connection. This is the reason we can appear to "have it all" on the outside and still feel so fucking empty and lacking inside. This emptiness signifies that we are lacking in the realm of feeling, of emotion, of fulfillment. That we may be putting romance on display for the *world*, for the sake of the "image" of romance. This type of romance is missing that connection. It's a bit like when we feel the pressure to plan something elaborate for our birthday but realize, in an uncomfortable dress and heels, with loud music and a bunch of people we invited to get the numbers up, that we would have much rather it was just our two besties, or our mum, eating our favorite cake and chatting shit for hours. That is what perfectionism feels like to me. It feels like a bodycon dress that's too tight for comfort. Do I look good in it? Sure. But do I *feel* good? Hell no. Romance that is a grandiose performance for others, for social media, and for other people to see we are *someone being romanced* isn't romance at all. It will leave us feeling hollow every time.

Living deliciously is about choosing what *feels* good, as opposed to a life that *looks* good. Romance included!

LIFE STILL HAPPENED IF IT WASN'T WITNESSED

Experiences that don't end up on social media aren't a waste. They are still sacred. Life lessons that don't get turned into an Instagram caption aren't a waste. They exist inside us as wisdom. We might pass it on some day to a girl we meet at a party who faces the exact problem we once encountered. Our wisdom and our experiences never go to waste. You are a collection of all the things that you have experienced and you, alone, are a worthy enough witness to your life. Just because someone else didn't witness the moment with you doesn't mean it didn't happen. It ALL happened. It ALL still matters. It is still important for you to take care of yourself and romance yourself, even when no one else is around. Your face still glowed in the sunset on the walk home even though you didn't get a picture. Your outfit still looked fantastic and brought joy to the people around you. The flowers on the table at your friend's dinner still brought love to the room even though you forgot to capture it. Your life is not wasted material, just because you could not adequately capture it on a camera or exploit the moment for further use. The moments you wake up early and don't time-stamp your story to let everyone know, still happened!

Whenever I fear that I'm not "documenting" my life enough, I think of the bin man who sings loudly at every time he collects my bins. No one is filming him and it's so early that as far as he knows, no one can even hear him. He just sings his lungs out and moves the bins onto the road one by

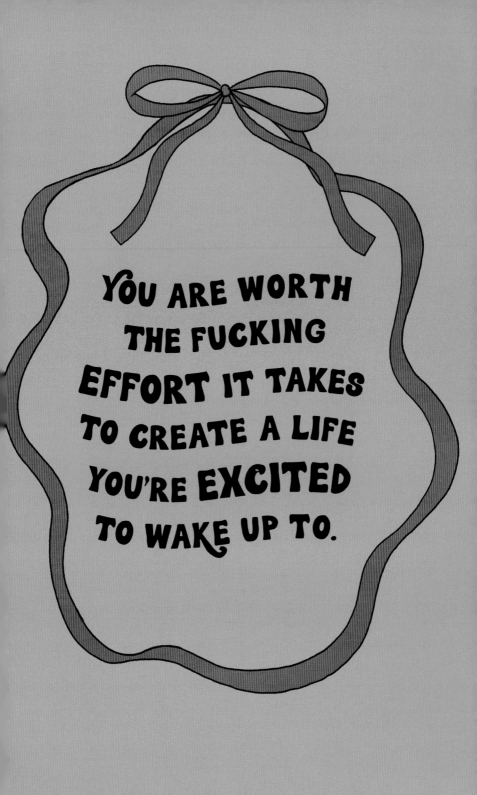

YOU ARE WORTH
THE FUCKING
EFFORT IT TAKES
TO CREATE A LIFE
YOU'RE **EXCITED**
TO WAKE UP TO.

one with a little dance. He does it for no one other than himself, to delight himself. Not doing it for an audience, or to prove that he exists, he does it because he wants to and, very clearly, it brings him joy. It's joy for the *sake* of joy. He carries it with him everywhere and we can too, whether someone is watching or not.

The less these moments are shared and the more they are done just for you, the more powerful the intentional action becomes. It becomes a way of being, not a performance.

Why is this sacredness of life without surveillance so important to preserve? I believe that we are collectively yearning for more thoughtfulness, romance, and intentionality as technology is increasingly reducing any challenge or friction in our lives. When everything has become so accessible that we no longer need to leave our homes to have food, conversations, sex, or watch a movie, I like to think that part of our ancient brains—so used to foraging, gathering, collecting, creating—is aching for something more fulfilling than the instant gratification available through dopamine-inducing apps. Romance is created in the process—and the process is being lost because we are delegating the process to someone else or to technology. We have not yet evolved and caught up with the development of our fast-paced society. Where does all of that energy go? The energy we used to spend on doing things manually? It leaves me feeling quite flat if I do not engage with this part of myself often. All the brilliant music streaming services, takeouts, and phone cameras have been built to ensure that the process goes off seamlessly, but none of them feel "romantic" because the *process* is missing. When we pay attention to a process—like reading a book, handwriting a letter, having to place the needle onto a vinyl carefully, or even watching a movie in the cinema—immersed in a dark room with strangers experiencing the same thing together—it demands more of our focused presence. It's a process that demands our undivided attention, which is what I believe makes these experiences feel so romantic. They require our care and full immersion.

When was the last time you gave your time to something that demanded your full attention, that offered you something in return and didn't leave you feeling drained?

REMINDERS FOR WHEN YOU FEEL IT'S ALL POINTLESS

One of the barriers we might experience in trying to bring about more romance and joy in our lives is the negative thoughts that arise in our minds because we do not believe we are worth romancing. Here are some affirmations you can use:

- I am worthy of these small, seemingly insignificant changes to my habits because my enjoyment of my own life is important.
- I am taking the effort to romance myself because it is empowering to nourish myself with a beautiful environment and experiences.
- Anything that I do to elevate my energy is not silly, it is a generous contribution to the planet that desperately needs more people full of life.
- I buy myself flowers because I like waking up to their smell.
- I am making myself a meal from scratch because I am worth the effort.
- My exercise is providing me with a better tolerance for life's stress.
- I am worth the effort it takes to live a beautiful life.
- I am worth the effort it takes to be romanced as a lifestyle, as a way of being.
- I am worthy of people that see how I treat myself and want to match it.
- I set the example of how I would like to be treated by how I treat myself.

Romancing yourself is about talking back to that voice, talking back to the unworthiness and making the choice to walk on the sunny side of the road, keep the flowers on the table, even when you don't feel deserving of it. *Especially* when you don't feel deserving of it. To be your own unconditional lover is to prove that you are there for yourself, not only when it's good, but especially when it's hard.

TIPS FOR LIVING DELICIOUSLY

Romance = creativity + intention. The world is loaded with potential. There are opportunities for romance everywhere.

- While some people see a pavement, others see a perfect sun-soaked spot with a view of the street to sit, watch, and make up stories about the people walking by. Try to seek out little spots, little urban "gaps" in the world for you to sit and ponder.

- Wear an outfit in your favorite color that makes you feel confident as fuck so that when you catch your reflection it brings you joy to see what you put together. The same goes for your nails. You look at your hands all day, so delight yourself visually!

- Leave handwritten notes of gratitude for people, whether it's service staff or friends. No one ever fucking does this so it goes a long way, and *you* can be the reason someone feels hopeful about the world.

- Pause on a walk. Just pause. Stop and notice a bird, or the reflection of the sun in a puddle. Stop outside a restaurant and look at the way couples and friends fill the windows by candlelight. You can use the beauty of the world around you to pull you in and anchor you into the moment. Into the NOW!

- Curate playlists for yourself to listen to during certain moods. I always listen to the soundtracks of movies I love when the surroundings match: the *Twilight* soundtrack in the woods or when it's raining, shoegaze music when I'm in Japan because of the *Lost in Translation* soundtrack, Mozart and Beethoven when walking the streets of Vienna because that is where they wrote. It brings the world around me to life. I'm not sure anything else on earth can make me feel as high.

- Observe people and look for beauty in them. There is romance in how they have dressed themselves. In every little decision they made for their outfit. So much of a romantic way of life is about changing the way you see things. NOTICE EVERYTHING!

- Women. Women do the most delightful things. Notice it. Acknowledge it. Women are romantics! An old woman who just finished eating her muffin in the café I'm writing in picked up the fork she used to eat it as a mirror to top-up her red lipstick. Then she put her lipstick back into her bag, which was a red that matched the lipstick. And her makeup bag was a leopard print that perfectly matched the one on her shoes. Women pay attention to such beauty on the smallest of scales—it deserves noticing.

- I really do take a scarf with me when I travel because it adds extra pink to a sterile hotel room. I am worth the romance of having a pink fucking room because it delights me and makes me feel cosy.
- I sometimes bring my favorite teacup and saucer when I'm traveling, because I want to have my morning coffee in a cup that delights me. A thick white mug doesn't excite me as much. But instead of complaining, I bring my own. Delicious.

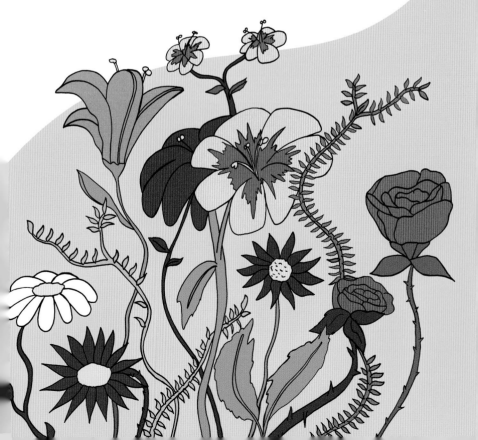

LOVE YOURSELF SO MUCH THAT DISRESPECT FEELS FOREIGN

I want you to fall so fucking in love with yourself and your life that disrespect from others feels *foreign*. I want the love you have for yourself to be so potent, so vibrant, so loud, that it commands everything that is meant for you into your orbit and rejects everything that isn't. The love you create for yourself must be so potent that it's impossible to even consider tolerating anything that might risk diluting it.

When you have been accepting *mediocre* as the standard for your life in love, dating, sex, friendships, work, happiness, you may not even recognize it as mediocre because it's all you've ever known. We can become so accustomed to mediocre as the standard of life. We believe that *this* is as good as it can get for us. We don't even consider that there are other realities out there. Not just for other people, but for us too. One where someone is dying to know how you like your coffee in the morning because helping to start your day *perfectly* brings them intense pleasure. Or one where a partner exists who respects your need for space, because they think it's hot that you have a life outside the relationship. Or where someone exists who you simply don't have to beg every day to love you.

Unless we dream bigger than what we know, the past is always used as our *frame of reference.* It creates that upper ceiling for what we believe we deserve. For example, if your ex was abusive and hated taking care of you when you were poorly, when the next person you're dating merely pulls a chair out for you on the first date, they look like a saint. You might even gush about it to your friends—*"They pulled out my chair and texted the next morning, they care about me so much!"* But all they did was pull out your fucking chair and follow up after a great date. I have heard myself gushing aloud about some of the most embarrassingly basic displays of respect I've received from people on dates before. But in reality they were nothing special, they just *weren't terrible people.* In fact, some of them were, it just wasn't as bad as the abuse I'd endured before. Without intentionally dreaming big, our poor, starving hearts can become so accustomed to unkindness that we cling onto any small gesture, mistaking someone's offering of crumbs for an entire banquet. But that's the trouble when you're starving – you'll settle for scraps off the floor. For disrespect to not find a home in our lives, we need to heal the parts of ourselves that welcome it in with open arms, the parts that still find comfort and familiarity with it because it reminds us of the people who hurt us, because it feels like home. It is not your fault. But it *is* your responsibility to level up your standards. We need to raise this standard by treating ourselves better. So that the love we seek is no longer a fiction but a *reality* we have already experienced, understood, and tasted for ourselves. We can command the love we want into our orbit—without ever having to beg, chase, and demand it—by *becoming* the love we want to receive.

When we don't allow ourselves to dream bigger and believe we deserve more, we settle for what we know. We start to internalize the narrative that actually it's us who's asking for too much from life and our relationships. We can convince ourselves that we don't enjoy oral sex because our partner never puts in the effort. That to be woken up with coffee in the morning isn't something we really need. That being told we're beautiful isn't that important. That laughter isn't that important. That physical affection isn't that important. Soon enough, every time we dismiss our needs in favor of keeping the peace in a relationship, we tell our subconscious mind that our needs are "not that important." They become swept under the rug, and we feel guilty for wanting *more*, for having changed our minds about someone we're with, or for growing and realizing we no longer belong in the relationship.

So, how do we get there? From tolerating mediocre, to accepting only what is delicious and enriching in our lives? Even when we have no proof that the things we want exist? *You become the proof!*

- You nurture a love for life that's so potent, that mediocre love actually starts to *taste* bland.
- You love yourself so hard, you can no longer lie about what you want.
- You extract so much joy from life's small pleasures that your ability to seek joy for yourself in everything around you envelops you in a layer of protection from settling for mediocrity.
- You change your environment and become the love you want to receive.
- You embrace your own idea about what kind of love you believe is possible for you, despite having never felt or experienced it before, by modeling that love to yourself.
- You do this all with gratitude for what you already have.

In my early twenties, I realized I had only ever received flowers as an apology after abuse. Accepting these flowers as a gift and having them on my desk became a symbol that I had once again been roped back into my toxic relationship, out of fear and guilt. I later reversed that relationship with flowers by making a habit of buying them for myself, when I wanted them. It was so uncomfortable at first. But it's become a luxury that boosts my mood, it's now an investment! Every time I look at them, it reminds my subconscious that I deserve nice things—not because someone is sorry they hurt me, *but just because they make me happy.*

Many neuroscientists have joked that the best way to find your dream person is to write a list of all the things you want in a partner, and then become them yourself. Romancing yourself and treating yourself with the same care you desire from a partner is so important because it sends a message to yourself that you are no longer waiting to be swept off your feet. No longer waiting for someone to show you how good life can get. Instead, you are showing YOURSELF how good it can get. You're no longer waiting for someone to prove to you that unconditional love exists. YOU become the proof that unconditional love exists. By loving yourself even when it feels hard. Even when you're annoying. Even when you make mistakes. When you procrastinate. When you're unproductive. In embodying love, care, patience, kindness, and generosity towards yourself and others, you start to put yourself in the position of actually experiencing unconditional love. You then start to believe, on a cellular level, that the love you want is possible. YOU. ARE. THE. PROOF.

BECOME THE SUN FOR YOURSELF

Can I even say I love myself, if it depends on the lighting? Or if there's a part of my body that I'm still hiding? If I punish myself for being unproductive and procrastinating?

Love yourself the way the sun loves everything. She loves you when you're spotty. When you're tired. Bored. Miserable. Unproductive. She does not shine on some and refuse to shine on others. She loves everything. Unconditional love means love with NO conditions. NOT, I love myself from *this* angle, I love myself in *this* lighting, I love myself *when* I'm productive, I love myself *when* I stick to my habits. If you take a moment now, can you see that you might have been placing conditions on the moments you've shown yourself love? Unconditional love must become the new intention for how you treat yourself. Because it is OH so fucking easy to love yourself when everything in life is going well. On the days you have your friends doubled over in laughter. When your post gets lots of attention online. When you stick to your resolutions. When you make good self-care choices. Or when you feel you meet the "standard" of beauty.

It is oh so easy to love ourselves when everything is going well because those are the moments we feel that we "fit" the ideal version of a woman. The "acceptable" version of ourselves. But can we love ourselves when we're "unacceptable"? Can we love those parts so much, we no longer view them as unacceptable, but deliciously human? Can we SHOWER them in acceptance? It's far more difficult to love ourselves on the days when we do not meet our own expectations, on the days when we make decisions against our wisdom, even when we knew better. This is why we must aim to become an unconditional lover to ourselves, the way the sun loves everything, the way a good partner would love your imperfections and champion you on. A partner that when you ask, "Do you love me?" replies, "Fuck, I love you *more* when you're like this, *because that's when you need love the most.*" Try saying that to yourself, in the moments when you do not meet your "conditions."

"JUST MANIFEST IT"

Manifestation is the process of creating something we want into a reality—a job, a partner, a lifestyle. But it is not just saying something to ourselves in the mirror and expecting it to just happen. Manifestation is not magic. Manifestation is just aligned action. It is action with *intention*. And it works. It has been proven with neuroscience that repeating actions over and over creates new neural pathways in our brains, the ones that, over time, become the most used paths, even stronger than the undesired behavior. Positive thoughts, when repeated, become beliefs. Beliefs that shape and change our actions, which then become our habits and create the results we want in life. There is no "manifesting" anything without action. We cannot merely hope for life to change. We must attract it with our actions, by making a fucking move and taking our desires seriously. This will prove to our subconscious minds how much we really BELIEVE in this better, more delicious life. We've got to get that mean, bully side of our brains on our side by showing it with our actions!

So, consider all of those qualities you desire in a partner and BECOME the person you want to shag! Because once you have given yourself a taste of the good stuff, it's hard to settle for less. If you can deliver the experience of delicious luxury to yourself, through the small daily pleasures of life—delighting yourself with everyday joy, centering your existence around your pleasure as often as possible—you become harder to control, less easily persuaded by others into lowering your standards. You become your own source of self-satisfaction. It is as though with each act of solo romance, you raise the bar of entry for others to enter your life. Gently, nonverbally, and beautifully. Whatever anyone can offer you becomes the cherry on top of the already scrumptious ice-cream sundae of your life.

STOP PRETENDING YOU WANT LESS

Choosing to raise this bar for ourselves may feel lonely for a period of time, because once we raise our standards, we may realize there aren't a lot of people around that can actually meet them. We might look around and see other people in relationships or with big friendship groups and be tempted to revert back to our old ways, because even though it's not what we want, we feel that settling is better than "nothing." This is when our old ways will become tempting. When we decide to stop reaching for what we want, because we get uncomfortable in the loneliness. But we need to hold on. Because when we have only just started to raise our energy and change how we act towards ourselves, our circumstances and reality won't have yet caught up with this internal shift. It will take some time to materialize in the external world. The longer we stick it out without caving into temptation, ignoring those texts from our ex, refusing to lower our standards, the bigger the gap between us and our old self will become, until it solidifies itself as a permanent shift. We quite literally become an entirely different person. One that cannot even consider being seduced into a lower version of themselves.

It will get to the point where we can no longer convince ourselves that we want less. Our self-worth eventually becomes louder than our desire for instant gratification. *Disrespect starts to feel foreign.*

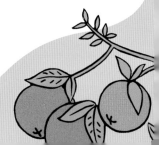

CULTIVATE A LOVE FOR YOUR LIFE SO POTENT THAT DISRESPECT FEELS FOREIGN!

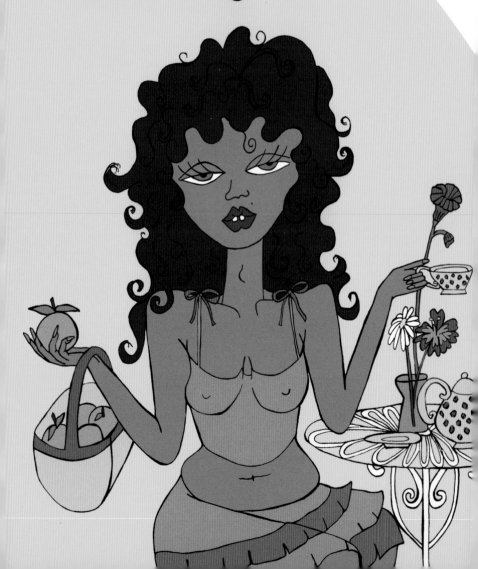

We realize our real worth in this solitude. When we can no longer outrun the things we're ignoring. When we give ourselves the space to examine what it is that we want next, instead of being in constant reaction to the world and accepting what's thrown our way, we begin to shift the direction of our future. We start to design it instead of default to it. When we are alone and choose to intentionally resist the temptation to numb or distract ourselves, we can no longer avoid the truth that we are unhappy, that we're settling for less, or that we don't think our partner is obsessed with us enough! There was a time when I was in a relationship and I was actually afraid of my partner going on holiday, because part of me knew that I would realize I wasn't happy with them if I was left alone with my thoughts. I would not be able to lie to myself in the silence. Sometimes, that's enough to know what we need to do.

Solitude is where you encounter yourself, it is the place you're always running from, the place where you can no longer pretend that you don't want *more*.

We will discuss the importance of solitude in depth later on in the book (see page xxx) and how to dip your toe into alone time if it's frightening to you, but for now I want to give you the strength you need to hold the fuck on. To not cave to your temptations to settle. To remind yourself of what you deserve. Even when the circumstances do not reflect it. Even when there is no evidence around you that unconditional love exists. *Be it. Be* the unconditional love you want to receive. We need to learn to sit in the discomfort of being alone, honor what we know, what we want, and take small steps towards acting on those desires. We can then create more fulfillment, more joy, more love for ourselves instead of using up our energy *convincing* ourselves we want less. Once we taste what it means to live deliciously, settling for mediocre simply won't do. Something I've learned is that no matter how good we get at pretending we want "less," the desire for *more* never goes away. If you want less, accept it. Be grateful for it, cherish and accept the life you choose. But if there is something inside you that wants more, something that yearns to expand beyond your limits, it will never stop taunting you. It takes energy to suppress what we feel and desire. It bubbles away inside us like a volcano waiting to erupt in resentment at the sight of another woman who lives the very life we are convincing ourselves we don't really want. Another woman should not be the battleground we use to fight our suppressed desires. She is just a mirror. You are not fighting with her, you are fighting with yourself. Remember, she is your invitation. She is showing you what's possible.

BEWARE: THE SELF-LOVE GOAL

The mistake I made when I started to intentionally heal was to make unconditionally loving myself into another goal to be smashed. The path towards it felt like another fucking hustle I'd taken on. Something else to achieve. Another task. My perfectionism didn't go anywhere, it had manifested itself in tightly scheduled journaling sessions I would feel intense guilt for skipping, morning routines I could not miss, restrictions about what emotions I should not be feeling because they were "bad." After exhausting myself trying to find the perfect morning routine, punishing myself any time I didn't stick to it, and eventually burning out from trying to be perfect at self-care (god, perfectionism really is a *disease*), finally the wisdom of that inner playful child kicked in: the beauty is in the journey.

Loving ourselves isn't a goal, but an intention, a direction, a slow and sustainable lifelong commitment. It needs to be a process and not an accomplishment. We will always feel like we're failing at self-love if we subconsciously make it into something we must achieve, quickly, before we're twenty, thirty, forty, fifty, before we're in a relationship, before the weekend of that big event, before the summer when we have to get our bodies out at the beach. The truth is that we are not projects, there are no deadlines, there is no urgency. Go slow. Go steady. One baby step at a time.

If the idea of loving yourself feels unbelievably uncomfortable and a foreign concept to you, I want you to start off by asking yourself these questions instead:

- How can I make my life and my inner world so beautiful and vibrant, that disrespect from others starts to feel *wrong*?
- Who do I need to become in order to be a match for the things I say I want?
- What would someone who loves themselves do in this moment?
- How would they behave in a situation like this?

We don't have to sit around waiting for beautiful things to happen to us. We are not victims of the present moment, we can become active creators in our reality. If something goes wrong, we can use our initiative. We can change, adapt, leave, evolve. Making decisions about our lives reminds us that only we get to choose what's next. Not our pain, not the annoying voice in our heads, but us.

Tip: Self-love doesn't mean saying "I love you" verbally. Words are not the only form of communication. We can show ourselves love by wearing SPF every day. We can run in the morning before work if we want to give our bodies the movement they need. We can get a good night of sleep. Nourish our bodies with food that gives us more energy. Stay home when we can't afford to go out. No one is going to step in and defend our limits for us.

It requires courage, it requires us to step out in faith and trust that we will catch ourselves.

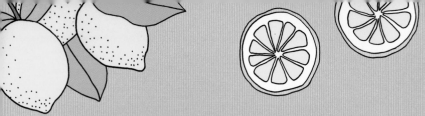

EXPRESS YOURSELF TO RESPECT YOURSELF

"Life shrinks or expands in proportion to one's courage."
—Anaïs Nin

A lot of us wrongfully believe that confidence is an innate quality, as though it is something we are naturally in possession of or not. We watch others and think, *God, I wish I had their confidence!* and wait passively for a future and "more confident" version of ourselves to be able to finally do the things we want.

But guess what? We will never, ever be suddenly confident enough—because confidence is built through action. Confidence does not just visit us one day and then "motivate us" into doing the bold and brave things we want to do. It's the other way around. We must DO the bold and brave things that scare us and *then* the confidence comes. Confidence is not innate, confidence is built through the proof we create in our lives, with our actions, that we can handle and overcome things. How do we create that proof? Doing hard things! Each courageous and scary action we take—whether it's asking someone on a date or going for a run for the first time—is a building block towards a future version of ourselves that gets to perform that action with more ease. We invest in making it easier for ourselves the next time.

We do not need confidence, what we need is courage. The fear of failure will always be there, and it exists in even the most confident people. The difference between you and your most confident self is the courage to go against that mean voice in your head. Confidence has to be built—through action, through repetition—like a fucking muscle. There are no shortcuts. If we forget to put the reps in, we can also lose it. It slips out of our hands slowly as we become rusty when it's not been put to use. We have to do the things we're afraid of doing, and it's these actions that build the muscle of confidence.

Sound scary? Not convinced that taking the leap and being courageous is worth the pay off? Let's look at the delayed and compounding cost of *not* expressing yourself.

- You build a resentment towards how you're living your life, as the daily inaction and the habits that are not in favor of the person you want to be pile up and you feel as though you cannot even rely on yourself. This lack of self-esteem is soul crushing.
- You start to envy other women who live and embody the carefree energy you wish to possess.
- You start to exist in comparison mode, where everyone is in competition instead of collaboration.
- You slowly develop "hater energy" for the people who have the courage to beam out the light inside that you're too afraid to express in yourself, instead of allowing them to inspire you.
- You attract a bunch of other people around you who are also afraid of expressing themselves, leading to more of the same fearful behavior, as the friends who become used to this version of you may hold you back from growing.
- You lack an ability to be happy for others.
- You lack agency in your life as you see everything outside yourself to be the "reason" for why you haven't succeeded.
- You trap unexpressed emotions and creativity in your body and drain your energy, leading to burnout.

EMBARRASSMENT IS THE PRICE YOU PAY TO BECOME FUCKING EXCEPTIONAL AT SOMETHING!

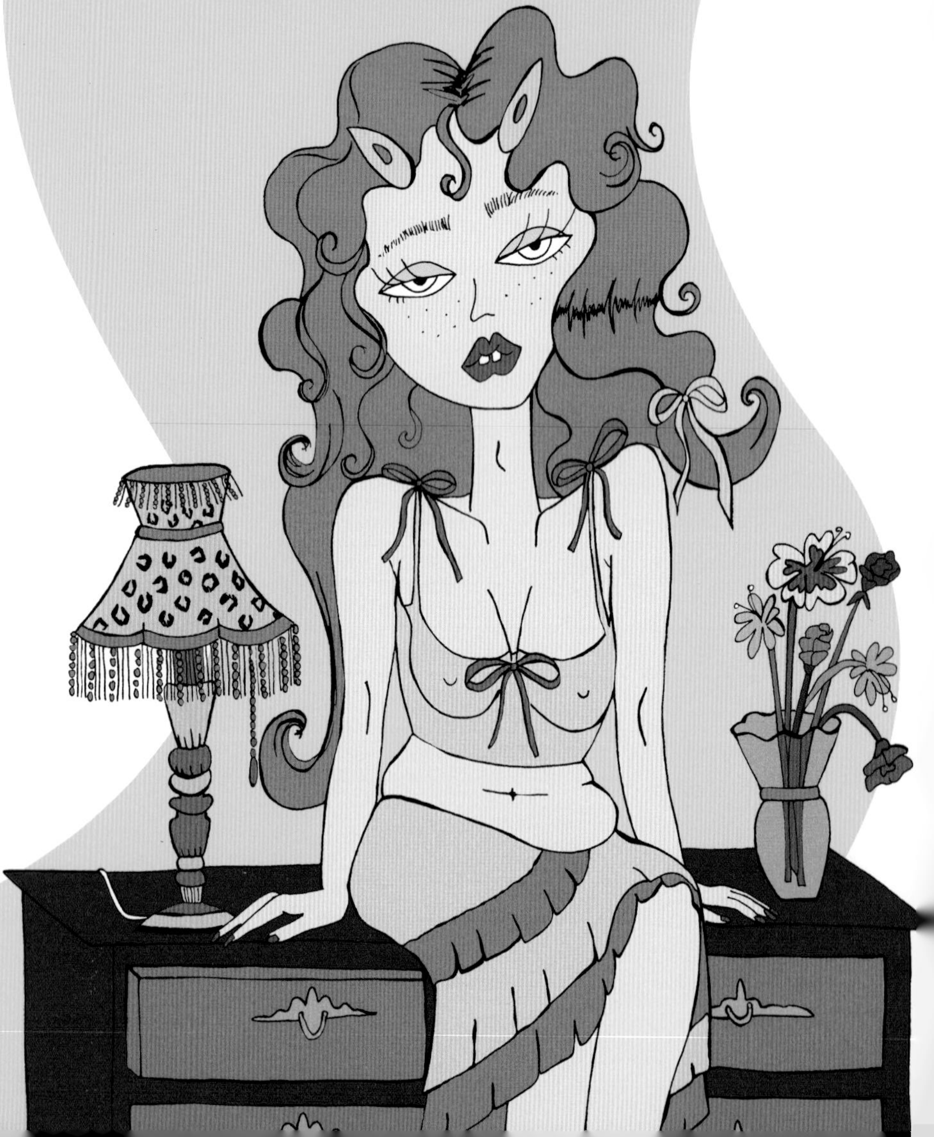

- You live a life that is the sum of your fears. Not your desires.
- You set an example for the people around you that acting on your desires is embarrassing. Fear is contagious. You spread it around you.
- You generate excuses like a MACHINE for why you haven't taken action, and your self-respect starts to decline in the background every time you do this.

Even though the cost is invisible to us in the moment, when we suppress a need to express something or act on our desires, the long-term effects are heavy and debilitating. Unfortunately, confidence is a "use it or lose it" situation. I had no fucking clue this was the case *until* I lost it. When I lost my confidence, it slipped away from me so slowly, until it was almost untraceable. I just found myself at the bottom of a pit of low self-esteem with no clue how I got there. I didn't lose it because of one big traumatic event, it was death by a thousand tiny cuts. It wasn't my trauma that robbed me of my confidence, but everything my brain told me to do afterwards to protect it from happening again. *Don't express yourself. Don't go out. Don't wear color. Don't trust anyone.* I slowly lost the courage to act on the things I wanted to do. Any time I chose to silence my opinion, not share my work, allow someone to cross my boundaries, skip going on a date, over-commit to social plans out of obligation, I was handing over the power of my life to others and my opinion of myself was silently declining in the background. Every time I agreed to something I didn't want to do, I subconsciously disliked myself a little bit more. Like a friend you start to lose respect for when their words and actions don't align, subconsciously this was the reputation I was creating with *myself.*

I started to dilute myself more and more, always choosing the safe, less courageous option. Consuming more than I was creating, watching others live when I wanted to participate with them, shrinking instead of expanding. This constant deferring of the courage to step into action led to a stagnancy in my life. The act of not expressing myself and not sharing my thoughts or opinions led to a slow sinking feeling I could not shake off. *How can I get myself out of this hole, when I do not*

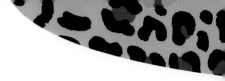

"have the confidence"? The shrinking of our confidence happens so quietly, it happens in small insignificant choices: such as choosing not to ask a question because we think it's silly, keeping a bunch of work in our room collecting dust because we're afraid to share it, or agreeing to things we don't want to do out of fear. We barely notice it happening. But if we don't express it, we suppress it. We push it further and further down and eventually, it takes root in our body. Fatigue, stress, burnout, depression, anxiety, and chronic pain can all be manifestations of repressed self-expression.

The more steps I took towards expressing myself when I was afraid to, materializing a world to match the vibrancy of how I was feeling inside, the more confident I became in my ability to not only create the life I wanted, but survive any remarks people might make about me.

WE DON'T NEED CONFIDENCE, WE NEED COURAGE

When we think of the frightening reality of the vulnerability required to express ourselves, especially when our self-esteem is low, it can feel impossible. But it's not. It is just a series of very small steps. Want to love yourself more? Start with doing your laundry. Then work up to carving out time to get outdoors for five minutes in the morning. Want to be more confident? Compliment someone's outfit. Tell someone "good morning" when you walk past them. It will feel frightening. But the challenges on our way to confidence EXIST to make us stronger and to toughen us up. The life we want requires a different person to be able to handle it. A more resilient person. A more confident person. And we become that person through doing scary things.

When we first try something new or scary, we usually stumble. Unsure if the ground we're walking on will catch us. We're human. So don't take it personally when things don't immediately go your way, or if your execution is not immediately perfect. Don't listen to the voice when it tells you, "I told you, this is a sign

you're not meant to do this." View
it instead as a *confirmation* that you are
making progress. Consider these mistakes as
your mental toughening ground, strengthening your
mind to prepare you to walk into future situations with
more confidence. To seize opportunities when they strike. The
trials and tribulations we face along the way are opportunities to
prepare for where we are going, for us to become stronger and more
deserving.

HOW CAN YOU ATTRACT THE THINGS YOU WANT IF YOU REFUSE TO BE SEEN?

When we choose to stay quiet, when we choose not to share our thoughts and desires, we stay in our comfort zone of safety. We're taught we need safety and security. We want a safe partner, a safe job, and a safe life. We call those who take risks "reckless" when really they are exhibiting bravery and a strong sense of trust in themselves. We must have great trust in ourselves to take risks, since it implies we have confidence that we have the ability to survive it not working out. Safe is good, but sometimes we can fool our minds into settling for something that's easy, that does not stretch our limits. Comfort fulfills our need for human safety, but it does not fulfill our desire for expansion. Ultimately it's a false comfort, because the discomfort is delayed. We delay it for a future version of ourselves that lives in regret of a life lived pleasing and playing it safe.

We often believe we need to be 100 percent ready to take the next step. Never just 70 percent or 50 percent ready. But no one is ever 100 percent fucking ready, they just have 100 percent courage and trust to put themselves in the face of the life they want. I want you to start thinking that even if you are 10 percent ready, even if you know a little bit of something, even if you've never been for a run once in your life but want to work out regularly, even if you've never published an essay but want to publish a book some day, even if you've never made a piece of art in your life but have a deep profound interest in it, I want you to act on that interest and make a commitment to take steps towards it. Taking steps towards our goals is what builds our confidence in our ability to change and impact our environment. We watch how one small choice we make shifts our day and the process becomes addictive. This is what got me out. One daily walk, one early bedtime, one hour spent writing and journaling at a time. It started somewhere small. You are capable of making the change you want to see in your life, and you do not need to wait to be fucking confident to live it! Live it and the confidence will come.

Have I convinced you that leaving your comfort zone is worth it? Going for that run, booking the flight, leaving the relationship, posting the video, leaping into the unknown, applying for the job? Leaving your comfort zone to leap into the unknown is worth the discomfort of pushing through, because otherwise you might feel the loss of the life you could have lived, years into the future, as the small moments eventually accumulate into years of inaction the way they did for me. The life you want is worth it. You can claim it now by making one move at a time.

HOW TO START EXPRESSING YOURSELF TO BUILD CONFIDENCE

- Spend ten minutes curating a playlist of music to listen and dance to first thing in the morning. Moving our bodies freely without concern for how it looks is one of the most delicious ways to feel embodied!
- When you hear a song you like and you want to dance, *dance!* If you can't do that, start small. Tap your foot. Wriggle it. Sway side to side. Do SOMETHING! As I'm writing this, Fleetwood Mac just came on in this café in Istanbul and my soul feels as though it wants to thrash itself around the room in euphoria. But my body communicates this with a little foot tap and a head nod as I type instead. Small steps! Get it out of you!

- When you see someone with a cute outfit, tell them. Never keep a nice thought to yourself. Even if you feel nervous about being so bold, this self-expression will build resilience. The more you interact with the world, the less scary it is.
- Post your content online without worrying about who sees it. Post the stuff that you want to express. Whatever voice you have in your head about *who will give a shit?* needs to go straight in the bin. This voice held me back for so long. But the aim of self-expression is to simply express. If I allowed that thought to stop me from expressing myself years ago, I would not be a published author.
- If you have a question about something, ask it. Do not be afraid of appearing "stupid." Do not be afraid of making someone else look "stupid" by asking them what they mean. Ask the question. Express yourself! Otherwise you might kick yourself, wasting energy by ruminating afterwards thinking, *I wonder what they meant when they said x?*
- Take yourself to a restaurant or bar—without getting out your phone. If that's impossible, bring your laptop or a book. Ease yourself into it. For seasoned self-daters, this might sound funny. But if you've never done this before it can be the most paralyzing thing on earth to even think about being seen alone in public. Dare to do it. If it feels embarrassing, bring this book. Take yourself to sit on a park bench if you feel you need to look like you have a "purpose." Just jump out of your comfort zone!

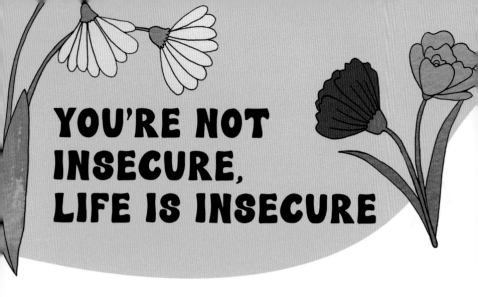

YOU'RE NOT INSECURE, LIFE IS INSECURE

We *feel* insecure only when we have tethered our self-worth to the things in life that are unstable and can be taken away from us—which is absolutely everything. Deep down we all *know* that things can't last forever, that everything is subject to change. Our partner's attraction to us. Our income. The love our friends have for us. Our pets. Our body shape. All of these things could change in an instant. We are not insecure, LIFE itself is insecure. I would say it's unfortunate that nothing lasts forever, but I'm an optimist—I think the fleeting nature of things allows us to love and cherish them more deeply. When we describe ourselves as "insecure," it is because we have an insecure *attachment* to these people, possessions, titles, clinging onto them for a sense of safety, which in reality, does not exist. Because even if we stay with someone forever, death takes us all. It sounds morbid, but it's true. Even losing a few followers on social media can trigger a feeling of insecurity because it plays on a tribal need to "belong."

We could say that "insecurity" is actually the fear of losing the *illusion* of security. Let's say we become official with our partner so we feel secure. Great! Then they start to mention someone new at work who makes them laugh. Our sense of self, if not tethered to something else within us to create a sense of stability, can become wobbly and shaken up by this shift in the environment. But if we have something within us to hold on to, a sturdy foundation of confidence to retreat to, our partner enjoying someone else's company will be merely felt as a wobble, not an earthquake leading to the total destruction and collapse of our self-worth. We want to get to a point where the tremor is felt, but we remain standing.

So what does being "secure" look like, if there is nothing we can truly hold on to and everything in life is subject to change?

Cultivating those *invisible* assets such as joy, love, confidence, and self-esteem within us will help us become less tethered to life's *tangible* assets—the clothes, the dates, the followers, the opinions others hold of us, all the physical elements of life that will inevitably change. Because when we embody love and feel love, we seek less meaning in the material things in life. We become our own self-sustaining divine fucking source of pleasure.

MULTIPLE STREAMS OF JOY

So how do we cultivate a security that cannot be taken from us? Something sturdy to hold on to when the tornado of unforeseen life circumstances blasts around us?

If you were to consult any financial advisor and ask them, "How can I become financially secure?" most would suggest finding ways to make multiple streams of income to ensure you are protected if one of them fails. They would DEFINITELY suggest having a savings account that you pay into on a regular basis to create a buffer of protection in case you lose your job or need urgent help. Security essentially means trusting that there is something to fall back on if something unexpected happens.

Just as a plane has multiple engines it can fall back on if one of them fails, we too need diversification when it comes to our "income streams" of love and joy! If we don't have a relationship with ourselves to fall back on when life changes, we will always feel any loss in our lives as a complete loss of *ourselves*. We might feel as though we're unable to carry on and crash. This is often when we have our awakenings, when we're at rock bottom and completely humbled by life, forced to see that something has to change within us. If we can cultivate a powerful, compassionate relationship with ourselves, when people break up with us, when things don't go our way, when something about our appearance changes, when friendships break down, even when our old ideas crumble to make way for new information, we will remember that we have something sturdy within us to fall back on. It then becomes less of a big deal to lose one source of identity, love, or joy. We will still feel all the emotions of sadness and grief, but we will have an inner sense of trust that we will still be okay. This is all a very long way of saying, "Don't put all your eggs in one basket."

The practices of gratitude, self-expression, and seeking moments of beauty that we have discussed in this book are the equivalent of accumulating wealth on the inside, protecting us in times of crisis. They all add currency into that invisible asset of confidence. They protect us from those future wobbles. Someone making a weird comment about an outfit is no longer a catastrophic blow to our self-esteem when we have our own opinions of ourselves to fall back on. If we can generate intense pleasure and awe by going for a walk to witness a sunset or even dancing to music, someone canceling a date will be disappointing, but is no longer perceived as the "end" of romance but merely the closing of a portal to it.

BITTERSWEET

I used to be opposed to the idea of detachment. I am someone who falls hard and OBSESSIVELY in love with my interests, music, people, and places. As a young girl, everything I loved became a *part* of me instead of being something I merely enjoyed. I could not fathom the idea of NOT immersing myself so deeply into something that I could not tell the difference between myself and the thing I was obsessed with. To place limits and boundaries between "me" and "the things I love" felt counterintuitive. I developed unhealthy enmeshed relationships not just with people, but with possessions. In an attempt to correct this way of being later in life, I started to close myself off. I thought there was something wrong with the part of me that yearned to connect, to be open, to love everything in my orbit since it was what had caused me the most pain. But we do not have to give up our love and openness. We can still be deeply obsessed and in love with everything we interact with. We just need to release them when it's time to go.

The practice of letting go allows us to enjoy things in our lives even more, since we are no longer trying to control them, chase them, or demand they deliver happiness to us. Detaching from them allows us to engage with life and our possessions in the way they were intended— for playing, enhancing, and relishing. We can enjoy them for what they are—the mere cherry on top, the decorative element to the delicious sundae of our lives. We can be obsessively in love with our lives and know that everything in them, at some point, will leave us. It is this bittersweet dance that makes being alive so fucking delicious.

Everything in life must come to an end, but that's what makes our time here so beautiful. There is a beauty in the knowledge that most of life is fleeting and insecure. Nature has seasons, for rest, expansion, shedding, growth, contemplation, releasing, letting go, letting new things bloom. We have cycles in life too. When we can start to appreciate the seasonality of life and how short our blip on earth is, we realize there was nothing wrong with us, but that it was our attachment to life itself that was causing our suffering. The obsessive, in-love-with-everything little girl is still alive and thriving in me, but she has slowly learned to let go when things want to leave her, and relish in a newly emerged truth, that it is making room for something new to enter, that she will survive the "loss," that she will never be abandoned as long as she has herself.

Life is short and bittersweet. The more comfortable we can get with breathing it in fully *and* releasing it entirely when it wants to change, the more we're able to enjoy it. What a luxury it is to love and be loved. What a flex it is to simply be alive. Love it as much as possible, relish in everything you eat, tell people the truth, be honest with yourself, live in a gentle yet urgent way so life's insecurity becomes an empowering reminder of how much we should appreciate it all.

We need to contain two contradicting truths: we are the only people who can change our lives, and yet we don't have any control over what happens *to* us. We can only choose how we respond to it. When we can slowly accept this truth, we can begin to enter a healthier relationship with life, in which we are not trying to control it or manipulate it to extract what we want from it, but generate what we desire for ourselves. In turn, we can start to shift our attention away from worrying about it being finite and invest it instead in the joy of being here, alive, breathing, now. Today. Doesn't that sound so much more fucking beautiful? We find that once we generate this inner wealth, the outside starts to improve too, as if the universe is now aligning itself, playing catchup with the way we feel. We can improve our lives from the inside out! When we recognize that we are the source of these creations, we feel less attached to them because we trust in our ability to create them again and again and again. What could be wealthier than an ability to self-generate happiness?

Most of us only realize the impermanence of things through loss, or when the rug is pulled from under us in a life-shattering event—like when a woman who is taught to identify with her appearance starts to age and realizes the confidence she possessed was conditional on her looking and being received a certain way, rather than something innately belonging to her. The patriarchal power afforded to women through years spent chasing beauty, is yet another illusion we grieve as we get old, put on weight, grow out our body hair, or undergo physical changes upon which society deems us no longer desirable. We suddenly realize the love given to us was conditional, based on how we appeared to the world and what we could provide. We can protect ourselves, just as we would by saving emergency funds. By creating a reputation with ourselves through action and gratitude, allowing that respect for ourselves to become an unwavering sanctuary to which we can retreat. Because guess what? If home is within us, then we are always at home. We always belong—in any room, at any event, in our paja-mas, in the ocean, in the bed of a stranger, on stage performing for the first time. We do not need to wait for external things to shift to realize we deserve love: instead we can practice generating it for ourselves.

Turning towards this inner world has allowed me to feel grounded even in the most destructive moments of my life, where everything was being ripped from under me. It's a lot harder for someone to fuck with our peace when we no longer rely on the opinions of others to know who we are. To know our-selves is to bathe in our delicious non-defensive place of confidence, quietly refusing to give people the power to alter our self-perception and allowing them to be wrong about us. Because we can afford to. Because we have inner wealth! But just like confidence, this is something we have to actively engage with and reinforce because *self-esteem is a valuable asset that can depreciate over time*. It is something we need to nurture and tend to on a daily basis. Other-wise, we rely on stable conditions to keep us happy. And life, as I'm sure you're perfectly fucking aware, is deeply unstable.

The next time you call yourself "insecure" I want you to correct yourself and say, "No, I'm not insecure, life is insecure, and I am struggling to accept the loss of control I feel in this moment." It is not possible to be stable and secure all the time. Life would be fucking boring without the chaos. This journey is about becoming our own anchor in life's storms. Finding it within us in the busyness of life, when we're distracted, numb, forgetting that our worth is not attached to how good our skin looks or whether people like us. This is the dance we all do in order to be free, coming back from the darkness each time to a more secure and steady place within ourselves. Two affirma-tions that help me to find the rock within myself:

- I am okay with people misunderstanding me.
- I will not try to convince anyone of my goodness.

Next, we're going to take a look at the many ways we can begin cultivating that inner wealth and make a fucking banquet out of our lives, through the practice of gratitude and curiosity. This is where it starts to get really fucking delicious!

THE ART OF BEING EASILY DELIGHTED

Master the art of being easily delighted and you will become one of the most mentally wealthy people on the planet.

And yes, it's an art. It's a skill. It's something we need to be open to, invite in, and seek out. There are moments of beauty to delight us absolutely everywhere. It is impossible to be bored when we practice viewing life as infinitely delighting. Which, IT IS!

I used to fear that my ability to be easy delighted by life was a weakness. I feared it contradicted the high standards I was trying to develop for how I was treated by others, that it meant people would be able to take advantage of me if I was so easily swept off my feet by such "small" things. But in reality, it's allowed me to create a life so full and vibrant, full of delights whenever I wanted them, that it protected me from the *temptation* to settle for other people's crumbs! It provided an untouchable, vibrant, and rich inner wealth that no one could touch or take away from me. It is my most valuable asset.

Gratitude has saved my life so many times. In moments when I didn't want to be alive, when the suffering was unbearable, at least I could go for a walk, watch a bird and realize how beautifully insignificant I am through its eyes. At least I could listen to My Bloody Valentine and be transported into a world that allowed me to indulge in melancholy and cry my eyes out. At least I could head to the comments section of my favorite songs on YouTube and feel connected to people who like the same things as I do.

At least I could take a deep breath.

At least I had this.

At least, at least, at least.

I will always have sunrises and sunsets. I will always be able to visit a park and witness the novelty of the seasons shifting, from the feeling of sharp frosty air on my nose to the first daffodil of spring.

The more I practiced the habit of searching for things to be grateful for— smiles from people, random flowers on the side of the street, noticing a moment between a mother and her baby and allowing my heart to expand as I watched the love pour between them—the more these moments appeared in my life. And the sillier I felt for ever believing that the fearful voice of my trauma, hell-bent on dragging me down with it, was the truth. In the most humbling way possible, I felt foolish for giving the voice of other people's opinions a home inside me, and the power to make me feel that my life was over the moment they decided to leave or hurt me.

But equally, I felt grateful to them, because life tastes far more delicious after you bounce back from the darkness. They were the springboard for my newfound gratitude. Life's small pleasures humbled me over and over again the more I found reasons to live, in absolutely *everything*. How could my life be over if there are still more songs to listen to? Cities to visit? Mornings to feel the dewy grass between my toes in the summer? Lips to kiss? Roses to sniff? Delighting in life's small pleasures ensures you always have a "reason." Your life is not over when they say so. Your life is not over when they leave you. When they hurt you. When they exclude you. When a business fails. When they ghost you. When you feel like you have failed at work. In these moments, you find something small that you're grateful for and you remind yourself: at least I have this.

At least, at least, at least.

Looking for these moments in my life felt like the opposite of being in a state of distress and rumination, when everything around pulled me further and further down. By seeking beauty intentionally, everything was pulling me further and further up. As though life itself was hoisting me out of the darkness. The effect it was having on my life was magnetic. The more I sought it out, the more I pulled it in.

Whenever I talk about feeling gratitude, I often receive comments from people saying they can't seem to feel it: *I can't feel gratitude, I'm depressed. I live an aweless existence, I can't see anything beautiful, that's the problem.* And to those people, I hear you. I've been there. In the pits of depression, it's not easy. But this is not supposed to be easy. And you are worth the effort it takes to lift yourself up one small baby step at a time to make your life feel beautiful again, from the inside out. Gratitude was never supposed to come effortlessly to us, especially in the dark fog of our minds that depression, anxiety, burnout, and overwhelm can create. Of course it's not going to visit us there. When it's foggy in our minds, the sun cannot beam through, the light is not even in our field of vision. When that fog visits, we're often numbed to the small, beautiful moments. But gratitude might just be the thing we can "use" to hoist us out. Sometimes when we can't feel any joy in our lives, it's because we're waiting for joy to visit us. We're waiting for joy to "happen." We forget that we can be an active participant in the creation of joy. Sometimes all we need is to remember that we can continue to search for beauty in our environment, as it gives us a sense of agency and confidence that we have *some* power, however small, over our lives. Finding joy becomes a quest we can set our minds on. The more we look, the more we see. The more the details of our surroundings reveal themselves.

STOP WAITING, START SEEKING

Gratitude is a habit. It's something to practice intentionally in small steps. It is a habit we must build, to create new pathways in our minds geared towards always searching for the beauty in life, even when it feels impossible to find it. To find a sliver of beauty does not mean to abandon our harsh realities, or be ignorant to the suffering of ourselves or others—to find beauty in something is to create an anchor in our life, that slows us down and reminds us we don't have to be beaten down and made small by the thoughts in our heads.

During a low period of my life, I stopped dancing. I stopped going for walks. Perhaps my body didn't feel safe to let itself feel free, perhaps it felt

SOMETIMES WE CAN'T FEEL JOY BECAUSE WE'RE WAITING FOR IT TO "HAPPEN" TO US. WE FORGET THAT WE CAN ALSO SEEK IT OUT!

unsafe expressing itself and being viewed by others. Whatever the reason, I just "didn't feel like dancing" anymore. But I slowly realized that I had let go of this life-giving exercise that used to make me feel so vibrant and full of life. I did not consider that the lack of happiness in my life was partly because my mind had convinced me I was "too depressed" to do the things that brought me joy. What if dancing was the "thing" that could hoist me out of the dark? What if going for a walk, even though I dreaded the idea, would provide me with the perspective required to realize my problems were small? So I decided to try, even if I did it crying and laughing at myself. During this period of healing, my life became a series of daily demonstrations to myself—through one walk, one dance at a time—that I would not allow someone else, or my fearful brain, to tell me my life is over. I did this by putting one foot in front of the other, over and over again.

It can be hard to stop our minds from chattering and even harder to separate ourselves from this darkness filling them. But remember, it is not you. You can disobey it. You can object to it. There is nothing wrong with you, darkness is capable of visiting everyone. It has yanked me down into the pit of apparent no-return plenty of times. But there are coping strategies we can develop so it doesn't swallow us whole. We can use gratitude as our anchor, the thing we hold on to in life's storms.

Being grateful puts us in a direct position to receive more beauty because it means we are widening our perspective, being open to seeing things we would have otherwise not noticed. The speed at which love enters my life when I am fully open to it is fucking ferocious! When my mind is not focused on ruminating, when I use the world around me to pull me into the present moment, love rushes in. When we are fearful or stressed, we become closed off to everything. We cannot marvel at the way the tiny segments of the orange we're eating burst in our mouth, or the sound of bubbles popping in the foam of our coffee. Not because we're "ungrateful" but because our awareness is too absorbed by our thoughts. The trouble is, when we stay in survival mode for too long, putting the walls up around us by staying busy, not going out anymore, avoiding intimacy, avoiding LIFE in an effort to protect ourselves from anything bad happening, we don't realize that *nothing good can get in either.*

Try something as simple as sniffing your coffee before drinking it to appreciate the smell, or welcoming the calming sensation of sinking into a hot bath. Gratitude! Complimenting someone's outfit. Gratitude! Smiling and catching the eyes of the cashier instead of tapping your card and zipping out the door in a rush. Gratitude! Texting a friend or your partner or your mom to say thank you for something. Also gratitude! When you intentionally incorporate it into your way of being, you will find that there is nothing this love does not touch. It becomes a way of life. Soon you will be saying thank you to the moon when it is out. The sun, just for rising. Your lungs, just for breathing. Gratitude really is infectious.

Keeping a diary of these moments is also a great way to keep track of the small things that make our lives feel juicy and luxurious. Their accumulative worth has a profound impact on our perspective of life, not just in these moments of pausing, but as it unravels. When we treat beautiful moments as things to be collected, walking through life like a magpie for beauty, we find that it is actually everywhere. A commute is no longer just a commute, but a scavenger hunt to seek things that light us up.

GRATITUDE IN PRACTICE

Finding joy in the everyday parts of our lives and writing them down has less to do with "scraping the barrel to find enough things to be joyful about," and more to do with redefining our definition of luxury to the point where we recognize that it is all around us. Luxury is in the eye of the beholder.

- Time without your phone is luxurious.
- The sun on your face is luxurious.
- Wearing comfortable clothes is luxurious.
- The smell of a sea-salt breeze when you walk past the ocean is luxurious.
- Birds chirping in the morning is luxurious.
- Opening an orange with your fingers and watching the zest squirt out as you rip the skin is luxurious.
- Feeling the soft, buttery texture of rose petals on your fingers or brushing them against your cheek is luxurious.
- Your pet's soft paw is luxurious.
- Being awake before everyone else is luxurious.
- Putting on headphones and watching the world go by around you is luxurious.
- The morning dew on grass in the spring is luxurious.
- The humid smell of the earth after it's been raining is luxurious.
- The sound of rainfall on the windows when you're warm indoors is luxurious.
- The warmth of another person's body under yours is luxurious.

The thing is, we cannot fake it. We cannot pretend to be "completely obsessed" with the beauty of stumbling upon a vibrant flower if it does not actually delight us. To feel that inner sensation of gratitude, to actually feel these small things as a luxury in every cell of our bodies, we need to shift the way we view life. To see the world differently, we need to get curious about it.

The bridge between negativity and positivity is curiosity. Somewhere along the way we learn to shut off our curiosity. We see things "as they are" and don't take the time to contemplate them more deeply. Curiosity is the bridge that can actually enable us to feel everyday moments of awe, gently uncovering and unfolding new meaning in the spaces around us. So if you can't

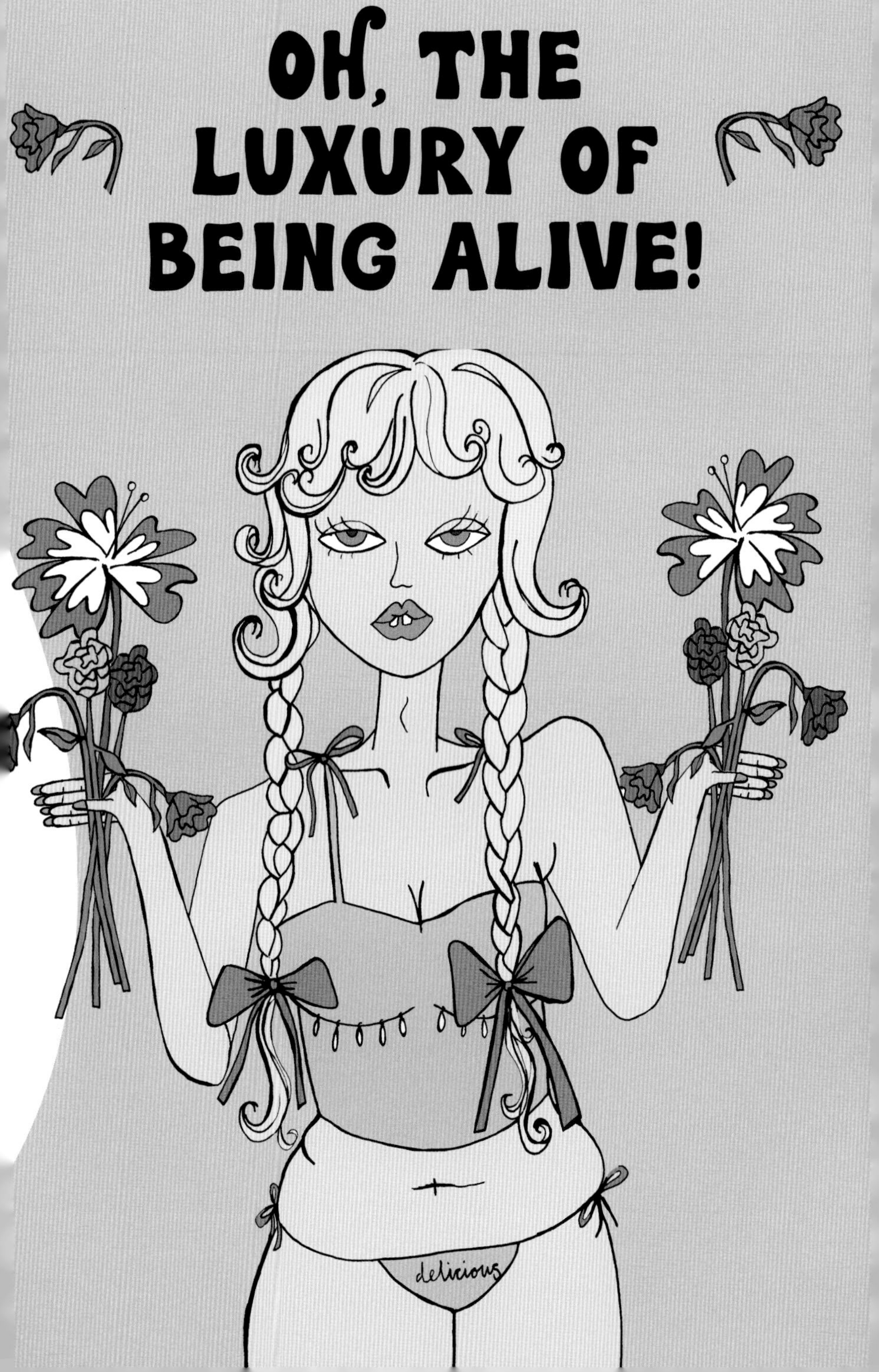
OH, THE LUXURY OF BEING ALIVE!
delicious

be positive, aim for curiosity! For example, if you feel nothing when you look at that flower, get still for a second. Let your mind wander. Where your mind thinks, *That's just a flower*, curiosity asks questions like, *I wonder who planted that flower?* Maybe you go over to inspect it, touch it with your fingers, delight in its texture. Maybe you discover a bee in its center, reminding you that flowers help bees to create honey, the same honey you had drizzled over your pancakes that morning. *WHAT? THAT'S WILD!* Curiosity sets our minds on a delicious frenzy of gratitude, awe, and wonder. There is so much more to the eye than what we see, there is a story in everything. This is how we allow the world to delight us. It is how we have more interesting conversations, make better art, become more joyful. We recover that childlike sense of curiosity and allow the world to delight us through it.

Stay curious. Never stop looking.

Practicing curiosity, in the way a child fumbles around the world in awe at the newness of life, can also give us space to consider that there may be something more, something deeper, not just in the world but beyond our current circumstances. Asking questions can give the events in life a new aspect—*I wonder what will happen next?* or *I wonder what this means?*—instead of the deflating idea that today's gloom is all there is. When we can only see what is in front of us—the job rejection, the bad weather, the date gone wrong— curiosity allows us instead to dream and consider that it may be leading us to something, trying to teach us something. What if being late for a flight can teach us patience? What if running into an ex can teach us to remain calm in uncomfortable situations? A great way to accept the things out of our control is through this curious line of questioning: *What is this moment leading to? What is it trying to teach me?*

WHEN YOU MIGHT BE TEMPTED TO LET THE GRATITUDE SLIP

We tend to let go of the self-care practices when everything feels good. When the sun's shining, when things are going our way, when we're dating someone new or make a new friend and the flood of love hormones pumping our bodies makes us feel like we're floating, we can think we're fixed. *YAY! I have been saved by something or someone beautiful!* We might skip our good habits for a day or two, or a week, or a month, to do something "productive" or something that feels easier instead. We forget the practice that helped us to feel this good in the first place. Sometimes, when we feel really good, we might feel like we've banked up enough gratitude to last us forever. Every single time I do this, I am humbled by a future version of myself who relied on me maintaining those practices, and is now struggling because past-me didn't. We can't use our rituals to "get something" quickly when we're feeling sad, that's what pleasure is for. Our gratitude practice isn't there to make it go away, it's a practice for a reason, because when it is done in the background over time, it's training us and strengthening us to be able to handle life. So the next time someone ghosts you, the next time you're late for something, stuck in traffic, your mindset will have shifted. It will no longer be an uphill battle to be curious, it will be the default.

We are human—we're messy, complex, beautiful, imperfect, and most of the time we get a bunch of shit wrong and act in ways that are contradictory to our benefit and growth. And thank GOD. I tried to be perfect and it was exhausting. It's much more fun when we accept our delicious messiness. It lets us love other people more for their humanity too. When we get things wrong, life slowly becomes one big cosmic laugh, instead of one big test to prove ourselves worthy of living it. I don't want you to blame yourself for neglecting your gratitude practice. It's not about shaming, it's about using something FUN to remind you why life is worth living. Never forget, at the heart of it, that's what it's about.

We can't exist here all the time, in that glistening delight. The ability to see life in this way and tap into that inner reservoir of joy will be blocked by stress, by life, by shame, by trauma, by distractions, by focus, by suffering, by comparison and negative thoughts. It is hard in these moments to feel delighted. But then, something in us remembers . . . *I can find something beautiful.*

And off we go, on our quest to find something to delight us. We trigger our curiosity back into action.

AGGRESSIVE AFFIRMATIONS FOR THE SKEPTICS

"Optimism is usually defined as a belief that things will go well. But that's incomplete. Sensible optimism is a belief that the odds are in your favor, and over time things will balance out to a good outcome, even if what happens in between is filled with misery."
—Morgan Housel

A lot of us feel afraid of embracing a hopeful attitude towards life and opt for the safety of cynicism. We mask it with an intellectual front of being "reasonable," but deep down we fear we'll be embarrassed if things don't turn out how we hoped. It makes us feel exposed and vulnerable. It's a lot safer to be a cynic. But optimism is courageous as hell! Being optimistic doesn't mean you are ignorant. It does not mean ignoring how things are, but it does mean knowing that it's worth sticking around to see what happens. Optimists literally live longer on average. If you can't be positive, you can at least be curious.

For the cynics who are afraid of believing "life is beautiful" or "there is joy all around you," I am going to offer a middle route. If you're a pessimist and want to adopt a more optimistic outlook because you know it's probably very good for your mental health, but the idea of talking whimsically and beautifully about life is giving you the "ick," try being positive in your own tone. Our positivity feels more realistic when it is expressed through our tone, our own form of self-expression. If you're someone who leans towards a negative outlook, try harnessing some of that pessimist energy when something good happens.

If something goes well in your day? Try saying, "*WELL, isn't that fucking TYPICAL!*" Or try, "Who would have fucking guessed it! Of course this would happen to me!" when the sun comes out. Or you can outwardly exclaim, "UGH! I look fucking fantastic!" and throw your hands up every time you look at yourself in the mirror. "Today is going to be fucking amazing because I said so!" By talking in this way, your brain believes it more, the message soaks in because it sounds like you. Try to filter your affirmations through your own voice. Whatever that sounds like.

By saying positive things in a tone that feels familiar to us, we can use the neural pathways created in our brains from the bad habit of complaining to stack our new habit of positivity on top. This might actually be the thing *that sinks in and yields results!* Because it doesn't feel fake or disingenuous. It sounds more believably you. Use your hardwired instinct to complain and talk negatively to introduce the new habit of positivity. Use your age-old habit of cynicism for good. Learn to delight in the world around you without abandoning your personality. When you start to let it in, it will reflect in your personality. And that is a very beautiful thing.

Life *isn't* beautiful all the time. We shouldn't pretend that it is, and doing so will only lead to feeling worse. However, in true optimist fashion, in the next chapter, we're going to take a closer look at how even being triggered back into our darkness and our pain, while it may appear as a hindrance on our journey to happiness, is actually the perfect opportunity for us to release it—unlocking room for *more* joy, pleasure, and happiness in our lives.

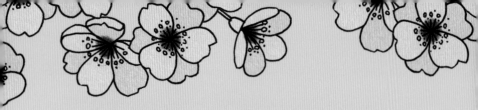

FORCED POSITIVITY FEELS LIKE CRAP!

On this journey of trying to love the shit out of our lives, there's going to be temptation to suppress our negative feelings in the name of "positivity." But trying to force happiness will make us feel like shit . . . because forced positivity is just self-denial with a spiritual makeover.

The last thing I want anyone to expect on their journey of growth is a straight path of constant fucking sunshine. Life is not always pretty! We have to untangle ourselves from the mess: walk off the track and into the dark wilderness of the beliefs, lies, and pain we have potentially for years been ignoring. Does that sound pretty? No! But life is about learning how to manage our negative emotions, not avoid them. One of the main reasons we embark on a journey of growth is because we want to stop feeling like shit, or stop making others feel like shit—or perhaps both. This is why we go through the difficulty of facing our darkness, so we can get out of our own way and heal from the pain that has occupied space in our lives for too long.

However, when we're striving to "be happier," we often suppress feelings of anger, jealousy, or discomfort because we view them as "wrong." But for joy to flow through, we need to release the pain we have been running from. We cannot keep pushing it down, numbing it, and escaping from it with our old coping mechanisms. Experiencing negative emotions is not a sign you're doing something wrong on your healing journey, experiencing "negative" emotions means you're doing a hell of a lot right. You are finally confronting the things that have been obstructing your path. You are now able to untangle those deep-rooted emotional weeds to allow joy to flow through. It is a sign you are excavating your pain and bringing it into the light to express, to alchemize, to create more room for the joy inside you to pour out.

Thank *god* for sadness.

Thank *god* for anger.

Thank *god* for jealousy.

Thank god for the emotions that remind us *where* and *what* our limits are: what is right and wrong; what younger and unhealed version inside us still needs to be loved more; what inside us is scared. Without these "negative" emotions acting as signals to help us feel and pay attention to what's going on in our internal worlds, we wouldn't have any communication between our minds and bodies. How would we know to slow down if it were not for illness and tiredness? How would we sense someone is harming us if we don't feel anger or sadness? Sometimes the emotions that appear "over-the-top" in a situation have actually been triggered by remnants of a past injustice done to us that we haven't healed from. There's a saying I love: "If it's hysterical, it's historical." If we did not have these emotional signposts of anger and pain, we would not be able to discover and heal these historical parts of old pain. Our negative emotions are a fucking gift.

Self-denial is something we all master so we can present a desirable version of ourselves to the world. At some point in our lives, we learn this palatable version of ourselves is what earns us praise, love, or approval. This realization, that denying a part of ourselves earns us love, creates a fucking habit out of it. Instead of being ourselves, we become what we need to be in order to receive love. This habit becomes our personality, which then becomes an unquestioned way of *life*. Until we get to a point where the façade of pretending we're "totally fine" is more difficult to maintain than expressing the truth and risking vulnerability. Trying to be the happy-go-lucky ray of fucking sunshine who never expresses a negative emotion is just another mental prison, one just as restrictive as patriarchy, controlling the acceptable and unacceptable parts of women's self-expression. To live a life expressing only positive emotions that please others is to deny half of ourselves entirely. When we suppress something, it doesn't go anywhere, we just push it down. We push it further into the roots of our bodies and minds.

When you're desperately unhappy and life feels bleak, forced positivity is like wrapping a pretty pink ribbon around a stinking pile of shit instead of acknowledging that it's hideous and that it needs cleaning up. Denial of your uncomfortable feelings does not feel good. Your brain FEELS the fraudulence when you try to cover something up. *Think positively? What about this ongoing battle I've had going on in my head with someone that hurt me as a child? What about the fact that any time I watch a woman thriving, despite knowing I "should" be happy for her, I am not, and a bit of me inside secretly hopes she fails?* The idea that you must reframe everything as positive—before feeling the negative emotions first—just replicates the same thinking found in cults. Suppress. Suppress. Deny. Deny. Brainwash. Brainwash. Believe. Suppress. Telling yourself "I feel fucking amazing" when you're literally ready to snap at the next person to ask you a favor is going to *feel* like a lie—because it is! This new lie acts as a barrier, making it harder to access that delicious reservoir of joy within you.

This is why healthy self-expression is the key to liberation. Crying. Talking. Expressing. Dancing. Singing. Walking. In these moments of expression, we release stored pain. It takes *energy* to suppress our feelings, so when we stop trying to push negativity down and allow it to release, the energy that was once being used to suppress it becomes unshackled, free to enhance the rest of our lives.

HOW TO FEEL OUR FEELINGS

As someone who has always intellectualized every fucking emotion and experience she's ever had—googling them, researching them in books, repeating my neatly packaged findings back to my friends to prove that I am *definitely, absolutely, completely in control of everything that's happening to me*—"feel our feelings" is an aphorism that has haunted me for years. I had no clue how to do it. My mind thought I was doing a great job at "healing," but my body was tallying up the suppression of my pain in the background—to paraphrase Bessel van der Kolk, "the body keeps the score." It wasn't until I physically burnt out that I was forced to face every emotion I thought I had

YOU DON'T HAVE TO BE A CONSTANT RAY OF FUCKING SUNSHINE!

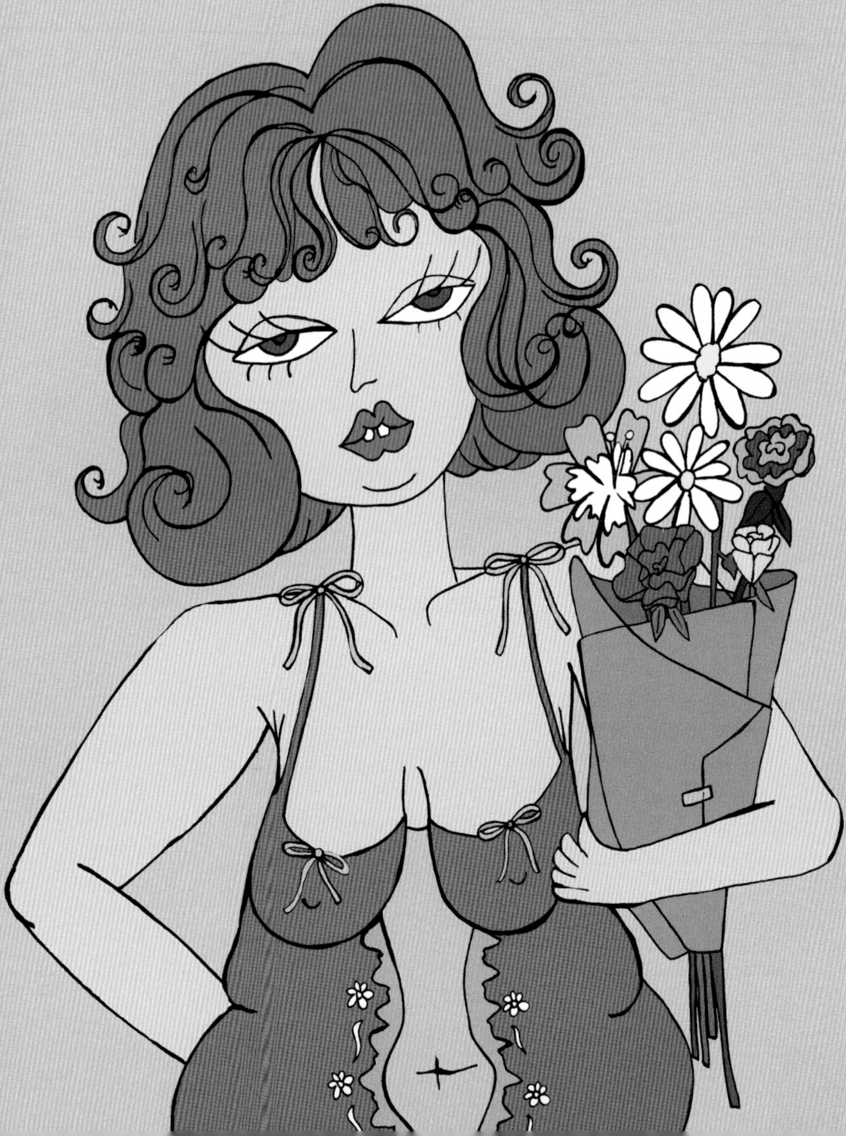

succeeded in outrunning. You can't outrun your pain, it catches up eventually. Every emotion I had been burying beneath dating apps, alcohol, social media, validation, hustling, working myself to exhaustion to make the "outside" look good, had erupted to the surface in stress, debilitating mental health and physical illness. I was forced to address the pain within. We repeat this cycle throughout our lives. We must constantly breathe in and breathe out the old versions of ourselves that no longer serve us. There will never be a clean slate; our bad feelings will be collecting inside us on a daily basis, we can only get better at regularly cleaning to ensure they do not become mounds upon mounds of stored resentment.

The first crucial part of being able to let go of a shitty feeling instead of suppressing it is simply noticing the shitty feeling. JUST NOTICING IT. Nothing else. When it feels uncomfortable and we want to soothe ourselves of this pain, jumping to intellectualize it, reaching for a drink, hopping onto social media, distracting ourselves, whacking out the dating apps, we keep the feeling inside us and it does not get aired. It starts to further muddy our view of the world. The key is to just witness it, don't try to control it, numb it, or endorse it.

BEING TRIGGERED IS AN OPPORTUNITY!

It won't *feel* like an opportunity. I repeat. BEING TRIGGERED DOES NOT FEEL LIKE AN OPPORTUNITY. You will want to defend, attack, call out, control, and stand up for yourself.

Every time I am triggered, it's like I become possessed by my past pain. Momentarily, my values take a sidestep, and this hurt and defensive part of myself lunges out to take the spotlight, the part that feels attacked and betrayed and wants to scream out, *"What do you mean by that?? Are you saying I'm stupid/ignorant/annoying/unattractive?"* This voice often sounds like a child—that's because it usually is the voice of a younger "me" whose pain has not been resolved.

The first time I actually noticed my triggered reaction instead of becoming it, I felt so ashamed. Who and what was that devilish and defensive *thing* that lunged out of me? In the clarity of a relaxed nervous system, hours later, I found that I couldn't rationally explain why I was so upset. It wasn't until I did some reading and introspection that I realized I had been triggered. When we do not feel our pain or acknowledge it, we can often project it onto other people's words and actions and see bad intentions that are not there.

The good news is, being triggered is an opportunity to practice releasing that old story or pain from within. By simply *noticing* that we've been triggered, we have the opportunity to take the pain out of the driver's seat and drive this shit ourselves. We just get better, with time, at noticing when the "pain" has jumped into the driver's seat. It shines a light on the parts of us that need attention. For example, *My partner is going out tonight without me* can be interpreted and felt in our bodies as *My partner doesn't love me or I am not good enough to stay home with* when filtered through the lens of our past pain. Even though we "know" better, our pain doesn't. That unhealed version of ourselves blurts out the same stream of thoughts, it echoes through us and cannot heal until we acknowledge it. Like a crying child that wants our attention, it can be irritating, we want it to stop, but it just needs our love and presence. By observing these thoughts instead of acting on them, noticing them as they arise, we can realize that our partner going out has no connection with the second story we have just told ourselves about them "not loving us." That this story is actually just the remaining sediment of a habitual narrative left over from childhood, or a past relationship. When that pain remains in the dark, unresolved, the wound gets hit and that story replays itself, over and over again. By noticing the negative feeling and the defensive voice inside us, instead of endorsing it and making it about our partner, we can slowly process the origin of this voice. Some therapists advise asking yourself, "What age am I right now?" to give insight into where the pain came from, helping you detach from the event that triggered it. We can notice the wound for what it is: old pain we have not yet acknowledged. In that moment of noticing, we are no longer possessed by the thoughts of our pain, and they no longer have their hands on the wheel.

Michael Singer wrote in his book *The Untethered Soul* about the concept of creating a separation between us and our thoughts. He writes that through observing these thoughts we can create a crucial "duality": there is "you," the noticer, and then there is the "thing" that you are noticing. It is no longer a part of you. You are not your thoughts. If your thoughts *were* "you" then it would be impossible to observe them, since a subject-object relationship is required in observation. This duality is life-changing and when practiced even once a day—by pausing or taking a deep breath to simply watch your mind—it can change the course of your thinking, which changes the course of your actions, which can change the course of your life.

For example, when experiencing anger, the thing you are noticing in your body is "anger." So there is now "you" as the subject and there is "anger" as the object. You have created a division, a gap, a space of sorts, between "you" and the uncomfortable emotion. This gap is crucial. You are not an angry person, but a person *experiencing* anger. When you pause to notice the anger, as something in front of you, instead of identifying with the anger and allowing it to make you say things you don't mean, or act out irrationally, you open a gap between you and the anger and create a magical little portal where infinite possibilities of how you can respond now present themselves. This "looking" and witnessing is the beginning of allowing the emotion to pass *through* you, not *become* you.

We've all got some shit we aren't ready to face. Some pain, guilt, envy, sadness, grief that we are trying to run away from. The only way I have ever been able to generate wisdom or joy for myself in life has been through *feeling* that shit. Not ignoring it. Not pretending to be happy. Not putting that pink ribbon around the shit to make it look pretty. That stinking shit has to be cleaned up before it contaminates everything else in our lives. Coping mechanisms serve us for a reason, and we do not need to feel shame for them. We should also not judge ourselves for the ways that this pain reveals itself. It takes as long as it needs to expose itself and release. Often in the most unlikely and bizarre ways.

I have released pain dancing on pub tables, feeling safe for the first time since sexual trauma to express myself in front of others, I have released pain in tears at a sunset, not just because it was beautiful, but because for the first time in weeks I felt *hope*. I have released pain in a morning stretch, in a wank, in an orgasm, in hugging a friend so tightly it was only then that I realized how badly I needed that hug, despite telling her for weeks, *"I'm fine!"* Healing happens in these small doses, in moments of safety when we allow our nervous systems to relax. In moments of *feeling,* not thinking. But we need to make sure we don't close off the portal to that realm of feeling by continuing to reach for things to numb ourselves or suppress. When we keep pushing our feelings down, the healing process never has enough space or enough energy to take place. The energy that healing requires is being used up in survival mode. Slapping a face of positivity over the pain, though a great tool to "power through" and survive for a while, holds us back from true healing and thriving. And soon, it's not just the pain you're blocking yourself from, no light can get in either.

Sometimes we need to take the long route to realize the answer was simple the whole time. Sometimes we need to see a situation from every angle, analyzing it over countless discussions with our friends, many Google searches, too many nights out numbing our sadness, to come to the resounding, simple conclusion, that the person who hurt us is a piece of shit and there's nothing we can change about what happened. That holding on to past pain by constantly discussing the event means we are still handing the keys of our lives over to the person who hurts us. That we still exist within their cage, living by their judgment. That we just need to let ourselves cry the tears we did not allow ourselves in the moment.

BOUNDARIES, BOUNDARIES, BOUNDARIES.

"Empathy without boundaries is self-harm."

Allow that quote to take a fucking *load* off.

Limits. I have them. You have them. Admitting we have them in the first place can be frightening as hell. Confronting the truth that we only have twenty-four hours in a day, only so much energy, and only so much social battery, can be uncomfortable because having limits reminds us that we are not perfect, but human. Perhaps limits in some ways can evoke this sense of failure. We attach so much of our worth to our productivity, and so to "admit" that we need rest often feels like a weakness, or a betrayal to the people we love if we cannot give them all our energy, all the time. Intellectually, of course, we know that we aren't robots capable of being in all places at once, so why the fuck do we keep pressuring ourselves to be? We all have something we are avoiding. A word that holds itself over our heads like a dagger, controlling the way we move through the world trying to avoid being wounded by it over and over again. Mine was the word "selfish." The word "selfish" was controlling my whole life. It convinced me that to take a moment for myself was the worst thing I could do and so I continued to please, at the expense of my limits, exhausting myself and afraid of ever slowing down.

Before we can get to living *deliciously*, we must brave it through the mental and at times physical discomfort of defining our limits and then relaying our limits to others. I've tried the other option, I'm sure you have too. Saying "yes" to absolutely everything because I was afraid of disappointing others, because the word "selfish" haunted me. Maybe your words are different. Maybe you're afraid of being seen as a "bitch," not being a "good enough partner" or not being "loveable" if you cannot overachieve. Perfectionism has different faces, but it always originates from the same deep-rooted place of trying to prove and please. It has led me to the worst, most exhausting periods of my life when I became physically and mentally debilitated.

HOW DO WE STAY FULL OF ENERGY?

So how do we learn to reserve a pool of energy for ourselves and our needs?

You are not contractually obliged to perform an expired version of yourself to make other people feel comfortable. Did you hear me?! I'm talking to the empath with no boundaries, the therapist friend, the doormat, the person who overextends and feels resentful towards the people in their life. *You* need to be the one to stop giving. It is not enough to moan to your partner about the expectations a friend has of you, or to sigh in frustration and hope they "pick up" that you're pissed off. This will not move the needle forwards in your quest to find balance. This will only further disempower you because you are still *waiting* for other people to give you permission to rest, permission to say no, to slow down, without asserting your need for it. We need to see *our* part in our own exhaustion.

When we enter into relationships with people, a dynamic is set pretty fast. If we meet people at a time in our lives when we're really miserable, or low on confidence, we might feel like we're breaking the "contract" of the relationship with them for trying to change or become more confident later on. To want more time alone. To start saying "NO" when we've always been known as the "I'll get it done!" person. We forget that we can renegotiate these unspoken "contracts" of our relationships through communication. We are not beholden to a version of ourselves that is no longer sustainable or authentic. We have the power to redraft the rules, state our limits, and say what we can and cannot provide. And the people in our lives? They have every right to leave! This is often what we've been afraid of all along, people leaving after we state our limits. But if we're exhausted and it's no longer working for us, the dynamic we're preserving is a fiction. It is not who we are anymore. It is our responsibility to communicate to people what they can and can no longer expect from us.

There's a question I want you to ask yourself. And you have to be really, really honest. Have the people in your life ever heard you say "NO"? I asked myself this question at the peak of my burnout, when I was enraged at the unrealistic expectations others had of me. I realized the person that was expecting so much from "me" was myself. I was still trying to maintain energy levels for relationships, projects, and roles that I had not communicated to people I no longer had the energy or even the time to maintain. I would sigh, I would commit through gritted teeth to plans, come home and moan that it was a waste of time and "I knew I shouldn't have gone." Yet I still went. It was me who did not want to assert my own need for rest and waited for my body to become so exhausted it said "NO" for me. As long as we keep getting things done for other people—confirming meetings, doing favors, and showing up—complaining doesn't count. Moaning is not a boundary. I KNOW! I'm sorry! But saying you're tired doesn't count. If you never say, "I can't do this for you," no one will ever register it as a "NO." It fucking sucks. It really does. We like to think others have magical powers and abilities to pick up on our resentment and inner pain. But they do not.

In order to reach the land of *delicious resentment-free bliss,* we must first brave the ghastly, stomach-churning terrain of setting boundaries. For women, who have for too many centuries been branded and labeled as givers and caretakers, this is going to feel like we're stabbing the world in the back. Our "boundaries" can be pretty bloody floppy. Nonexistent. They flow with whatever the people we love, or even strangers, want from us. They can be so dependent on others' needs that we're afraid to set them for ourselves, to define what it is that *we* want. So much so that we avoid setting them altogether and remain exploitable. This in turn causes us to become resentful, as we watch our lives take the shape of other people's preferences. We rob the relationships in our lives of the intimacy that is created by honest communication. There's always a fear that by telling someone you love that they've made you uncomfortable, or that you actually need the morning to yourself, they might think you don't care about them and feel rejected. This fear of "rejecting" them immobilizes us. So instead, we fucking reject *ourselves.*

When you're a people-pleaser, other people's innocent requests can feel like "demands." We might complain about all the things we "have to do" without realizing that we don't have to do them at all, and that WE were the ones who committed to doing them. A simple affirmation to repeat when people ask things of us is: "This is a request, I am allowed to accept or decline."

ENERGETIC BOUNDARIES

The truth is, boundaries are about you, not other people. The only thing you can actually control in this life is yourself. So once you've stated a boundary, you are ALSO responsible for sticking to it with your actions. Not texting back. Not caving into guilt and helping someone after you said you couldn't. These are what I like to call *"energetic boundaries,"* where we don't even have to announce we won't be doing something, again … and again … we just state it and don't do it. After years of explaining why you won't do something, or "tolerate" something, your actions are actually the things that show someone what you will and won't accept. You can shift people's expectations of you by refusing to stress about the way people behave or how many favors they ask (out of your control) and instead focusing on what you answer to (in your control). Have you told your partner for years … and years … that you're fed up with them belittling you in front of their friends? Your words might let them know that you're hurt, but after years of them continuing to hurt you, your actions tell them that you will stay no matter what. They don't believe there are consequences for belittling you, so they continue to do it. A friend sending you multiple texts about nonurgent issues? Get back to them when you are free—I'm sure they don't even expect you to get back as quickly as you put the pressure on yourself to do. You teach people how to treat you. You are not contractually obliged to be the same person you were when you met. You get to rewrite the contract. Act differently. The rules will change. And you will take a step closer towards a life that has more room for you to breathe, to design it for yourself instead of defaulting to what everyone else wants of you.

I have had to reverse-engineer years of saying "yes" to everything and doing everything asked of me by setting energetic boundaries. An energetic boundary could be not replying to emails on the weekends, even if your boss contacts you. Your boss might not stop, but that doesn't mean you have to reply. You can control how much you let these things invade your life by how you respond. Most people respond to actions, not just words. You can stop people from taking the piss by refusing to act in the way they want you to. Teach people that you are unexploitable by not allowing them to exploit you. Get used to disappointing other people's need for instant gratification. *Be okay with disappointing others, if the alternative is disappointing yourself.*

Something I have been trying to unlearn from my perfectionism is a false sense of urgency. Most of the time, there is actually no rush—things can get done in the same amount of time, with more quality, if I choose to slow down. Scrubbing myself hurriedly in the shower. Putting my shoes on quickly. Feeling pressure to be immediately productive in the morning. Brushing my hair in a panic. When I catch myself in a hurry, I ask myself, *why am I in a rush?* There is no rush. The energy of "rushing" means we can go a million miles an hour in the wrong direction without checking in to see if our desires have changed. It can prevent us from a more intentional way of living.

But where is this urgency coming from? Is it outside us, or within us? Is this time pressure real, or being manu-factured? Sometimes the reason we feel rushed is

YOUR ABILITY
TO CREATE A
DELICIOUS LIFE
IS DETERMINED
BY HOW OFTEN
YOU'RE WILLING
TO TRANSCEND
YOUR FEARS!

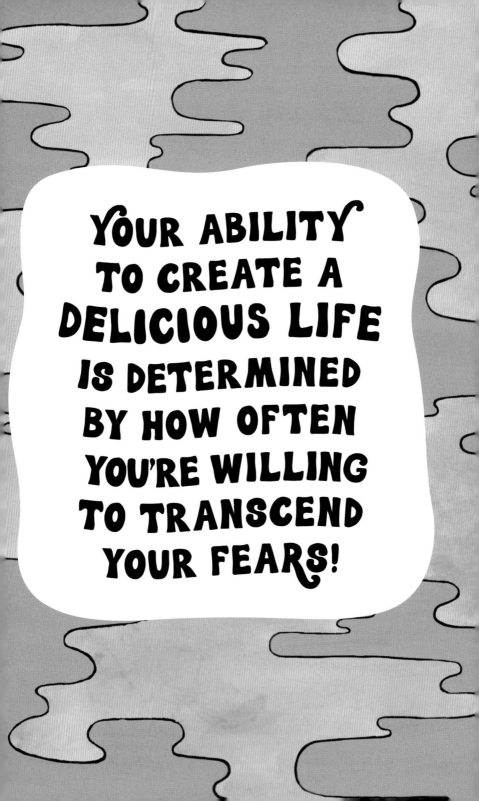

because someone is using a false sense of urgency to create a feeling of time scarcity, forcing us to do what they want. Ask yourself, is it really that urgent? Settle your nervous system. Take a deep breath. You can always check in with yourself. Does this thing actually need to be solved so quickly? If it does, can you try to do it calmly? Sometimes it's not about slowing down, but to simply change the state you are in.

Saying "no" or "that doesn't work for me" —especially when we love someone or hold them in high regard—can feel like holding on to a pole in the middle of a tornado. Braving the shit storm and waiting for the emotional turmoil of guilt and shame to pass is the key. If we let go and we revoke the boundary out of guilt, we abandon our limits and get whisked away into their request. Holding on offers us the freedom from being controlled by our own emotional terrorism. Normally it does not initially feel *good* to set boundaries, despite them being very good *for* us. You're going to feel like a bitch! You just will. Sit with the discomfort, focusing on the freedom it will afford you afterwards. Your rest is your responsibility. Rise to it.

SAYING "NO" CREATES MORE ROOM FOR "FUCK YES!"

Un-exhausting myself and weaning myself off the drug of external approval has taken me a very long time. Why? Because I was trying to have my goddamn cake *and* eat it too. I thought that I could set boundaries *and* not disappoint anyone. I thought I could honor my need for rest *and* still produce as much work as before. I thought I could be more playful and spontaneous while still secretly striving to be perfect. I wanted to express myself fully *and* not receive any criticism. But in order to achieve something, we have to sacrifice something. We cannot hope for change and *stay the same*.

WOW! SETTING BOUNDARIES HAS MADE MY LIFE SO FUCKING PEACEFUL!

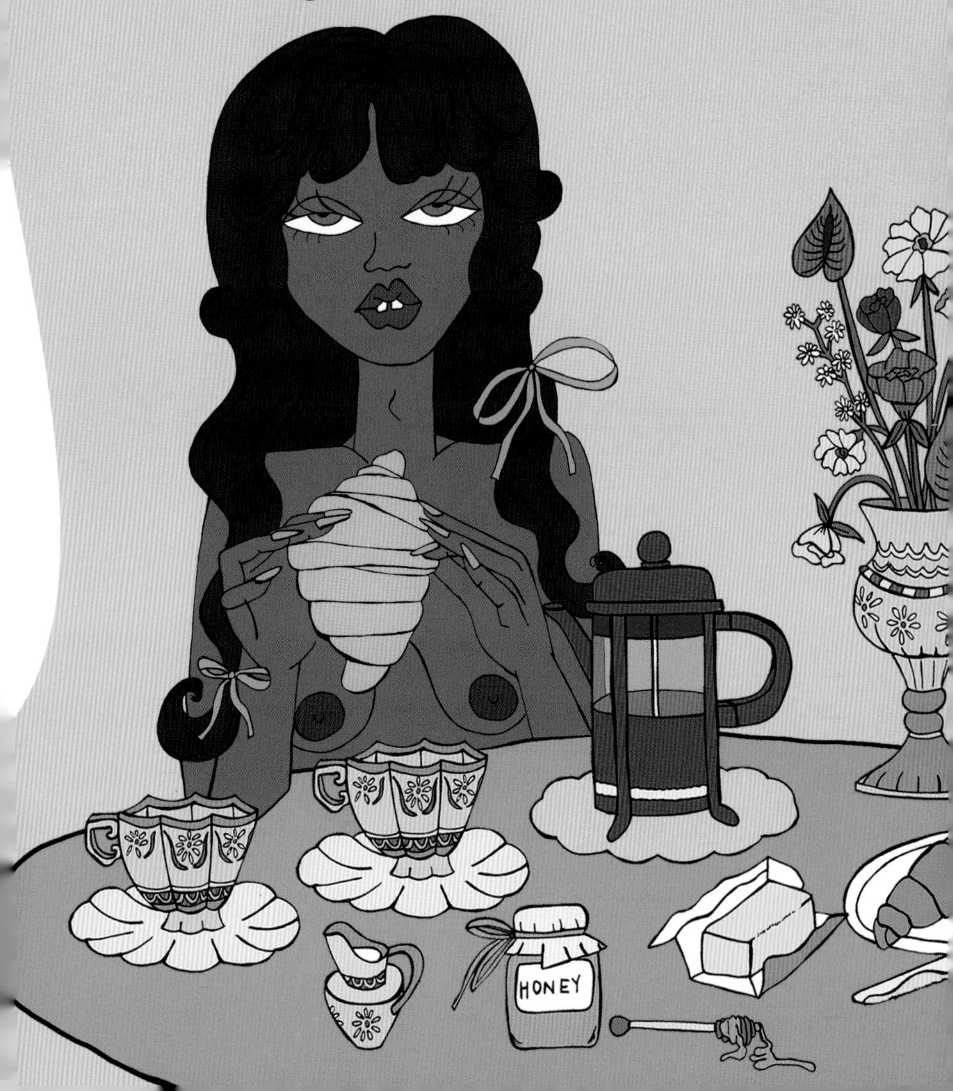
HONEY

The key is learning how to stand your ground, say "NO" even when it's uncomfortable. It doesn't mean you've done anything wrong. You're not in trouble. Let it pass. It's finally time to take other people's desires off the pedestal and replace them with your own. Put *your* desires on a fucking pedestal and worship the shit out of them! How wild to think that most of us have never, EVER, done this. I want you to get so turned on at the idea of the woman you could become if you started to release the energy tied up in pleasing others. What will that new source of fuel do to your life?! Where might that energy go and who might you become in a year, two, three, or four as a result of it?

If you brave the discomfort of saying "NO," you get to say "FUCK YES" to something else. In canceling that plan, you get to say "FUCK YES" to that good night of sleep. In saying "NO" to scrolling for another hour on social media, you get to say "FUCK YES" to calling your mom, or doing something that actually fills you up and doesn't drain you in the process. You're not "missing out." Not ever. You just gain something *else* in return. Brené Brown, who researches shame, found that the one thing compassionate people have in common is "boundaries of steel." The people able to be most generous to others are those who guard their own limits and capacity diligently, treating their energy as the precious asset it is. "Compassionate people ask for what they need. They say no when they need to, and when they say yes, they mean it. They're compassionate *because* their boundaries keep them out of resentment."

I am slowly letting go of striving to be productive, perfect, pretty. I want to be known as alive, compassionate, generous, and present—and that shit requires *boundaries*. Ironically, the beauty, creativity, and enthusiasm this generates is astronomical. It is not something you can buy in a bottle. There is nothing more radiant than a person who is alive in their own body. No one kinder than a person who has taken responsibility for their rest and is, as a result, completely free of resentment. Fear is a great motivator, but it is not a sustainable fuel and it will have us chasing the wrong things. Glowing from the inside *out* by protecting our energy, instead of perfecting the outer shell of our lives by pleasing, ironically allows the "outside" to shift in a way that we no longer desire the things we once sought acceptance from. They become fun. They become additional. Dressing up is no longer a thing we do to prove ourselves, but to decorate ourselves and have fun. Having to help others is no longer a burden, but becomes something we're excited to generously pour into. When we are already "full" we start to approach these things with a healthier attachment, no longer relying on them for a sense of self because we already have it. It is from this abundant place of compassion that we get to enjoy our lives properly, instead of living with the fear that every interaction is a test of our worthiness.

In order to become unexploitable, we must say "yes" when we fucking mean it and say "NO" whenever we need to. We must sit in the silence after we set boundaries and allow the other person to be displeased with us if that's how they feel, without trying to change our boundary. Like playing a mean game of poker, never fold to someone else's bluff. Their feelings do not call for you to change your limits or give in. Just as you are entitled to set your boundaries, they are entitled to have a reaction. Let them have it.

Say "no" to them and "yes" to yourself. Trust that it will help you become the joyful person that you (and the people in your life) deserve.

LIFE'S TOO SHORT TO PLAY IT COOL

I was always told that I was "too much." Too intense. Too sensitive. But I have come to fucking ADORE these things about myself. They are my superpower. These are the parts of me that have survived shame! It is so fucking hard to hold on to our enthusiasm in this world without replacing it with a desire to be "cool." To hold on to our ability to be ourselves against the friction of judgment from other people. To resist the cage of cool and embrace the shit you love, whether or not it's validated by anyone else. We collectively shame the femininity and vulnerability inherent in the expression of enthusiasm in anyone, regardless of their gender.

There is a subtle flavor of patriarchy in how the vulnerable act of expressing joy, regardless of who embodies it, is seen as *cringey and embarrassing*. The way that any vibrant expression of enthusiasm, awe, curiosity, and wonder—all beautiful qualities that make life worth living—are often called *"cringey"* in women and *"weak"* in men. As though the expression of delight on our faces is something we should be embarrassed by. We all shame this childlike "feminine" energy within ourselves and *praise* the "masculine" energy—the structure, productivity, work, planning, logic, numbers, statistics. We tend to discard anything that is intuitive or playful and belongs to the invisible realm of feeling, because it is intangible and we cannot see it.

During the process of writing this book, I've been thinking about the word "cringe" a lot. The fact that we are reluctant to express ourselves and display joy on our faces is a result of the collective suppression of the traits deemed "too feminine" and vulnerable under patriarchy. It's not just men, but women too who can experience a suppression of femininity. Caged in by coolness. Detached from delight. HOW BORING! How bland! Playing it "cool" is the seductive trap that prevents us from being delighted and moved by life. Most of us first expressed a sense of delight and curiosity in childhood, asking questions about everything and being amazed at the world. But all too soon we learned that it is embarrassing and something to be ashamed of. This passion and enthusiasm, often described as "theater kid energy," receives negative reactions and shaming from others, we learn to replace it with a detached nonchalance as a form of protection, the more stoic traits that are praised under patriarchy and shield us from vulnerability. *When and how did it become cool to be so numb?*

Most people can only recall having this much enthusiasm for life as a distant memory. But occasionally in adulthood we might feel that enthusiasm in witnessing a sunrise or a beautiful piece of art or music that silences our minds in awe. We allow the joy to express itself over our faces and for a split second we are unaware of how we look as we revel in the joy of being alive, until . . . someone walks past. We drop the smile. Clear our throats. Pretend we were squinting at something. Stop tapping our feet to the music. Stop smiling. What *is* that? That's cringe. You're cringing at yourself. Because joy, awe, curiosity are vulnerable expressions of that childlike feminine energy we have all been shamed from expressing. This is particularly an issue for men, whose sense of identity under patriarchy relies on and is built upon *avoiding* being perceived as feminine.

Men do it to men: If a man expresses that he cannot physically do something, he's called *a pussy.*

Men do it to women: If a woman speaks about her intuition, she's told *she's away with the fairies* or has her intuition dismissed with "logic."

Men do it to themselves: When their emotions take over, they bottle up their sadness and repeat the doctrine told to them by their fathers or other men—*Don't cry.*

Women do it to men: *He's not man enough. I need a man that isn't weak.*

Women do it to women: *God, she's a bit … much isn't she? I'm not like her, I'm a chill girl who doesn't get feelings.*
Women do it to themselves: *I'm too much. I'm too intense. I'm over sensitive.*

We cannot fucking stand this earnest expression and vulnerability in any-one, regardless of gender, it's like we don't know what to do with it. Even in women, we only like an expression of femininity when it services men's desires: submissive, small, and easily controlled. A femininity that is wild, childlike, expansive, and passionate is too complex to control and tame, it exists outside what's considered desirable and so we diminish it. We call it irrational.

When a girl is called "one of the boys" it's a compliment that will boost her ego because masculinity is "cool." But if a boy is called "one of the girls," it's an insult that can have his "man card" revoked and his sexuality called into question. Misogyny cannot be merely defined as the hatred of women, but as a cultural disgust of femininity and its vulnerable forms of expression, regardless of whoever possesses it. It's an undermining of femininity, a de-valuing of it as something that is weak, frivolous, silly. The truth is, a whole human being is one that has integrated all of their parts. That is where heal-ing happens. It cannot happen when we're fragmented, splitting half of our emotional world away out of shame.

I think I might have been subconsciously trying to avoid someone saying I'm "too much" or "too sensitive" my whole adult life, and it was precisely this fear that has prevented me from getting high on the curiosity I used to feel as a child. It has stopped me in the past from being enthusiastic, from loving the shit out of the things I adore whether people think that they're cool or not. I built walls around that part of myself, trying to protect this joyful and childish part of me that had been criticized and laughed at before. I didn't ever want her to get hurt again. I did not want her to be called *cringe*.

YOUR HAPPIEST SELF IS ALSO YOUR CRINGIEST SELF. JUST FUCKING EMBRACE IT!

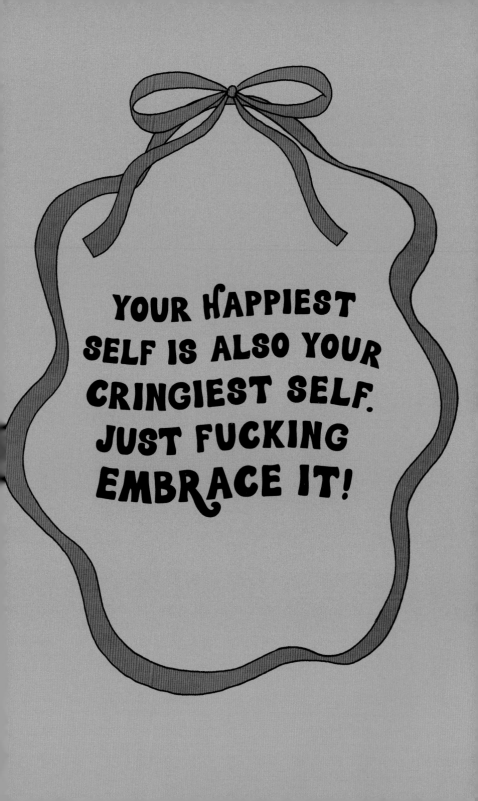

CRINGE!

To talk further about cringe, we need to properly define it. Because as long as we don't define it, we can kind of "get away" with abusing the word to shame other people. *She's so cringey! Did you see her outfit?* What if the cringe and embarrassment we see in others belongs to us? What if they're not cringey, what if something within *us* has cringed? What if the cringe is *ours*?

Let's take a closer look at the qualities that normally make up something we class as "cringey":

- Passion
- Trying really hard at something
- Being earnest
- Experiencing childlike awe
- Vulnerability
- Optimism
- Self-expression that we perceive to be "unaware" of social norms
- Self-promotion
- Ambition
- THEATER KID ENERGY!
- Expressing our emotions

Isn't it ironic that these are all the key ingredients to living a delicious and open life?

No, really. Read that list again. How are we supposed to experience *any* joy in our lives without these things? These are not things to be embarrassed by; these are all the emotions and expressions that, when embraced without shame, allow us to be touched by life. These are all the openings that allow us to be delighted! I've wondered for a while what it is that makes us "cringe." We can normally point to actions, behaviors, and things that give us this inner feeling that could be described as a wriggly, writhing discomfort at someone else's display of vulnerable self-expression we consider to be "embar-

rassing." But I have noticed
that I cringe less when I am on my
own. That this cringe feeling is intensified when
I'm around others. We often feel we need to outwardly
"express" our cringe among other people—with a snicker, a
laugh, or by overtly saying "cringe!" under our breath to show
that we tribally "belong" and adhere to the codes of behavior that
we've been taught to place ourselves within. But what is the string
that connects all of these things we cringe at? What is it that makes one
person cringe at someone dancing, and another relish in awe at the sight of
someone happy to be alive in their body?

I believe we cringe at the things we see in others we have repressed within
ourselves, whether it is something we were told not to do as a child, or learned
to avoid as an adult. The things we cringe at are ACTUALLY revealing the
parameters of our own social conditioning, the lines inside ourselves that we,
personally, have been taught not to cross, the things that we have learned to
view as socially unacceptable. The things we "cringe" at appear to be anything
that exists beyond our own, personal comfort zone of self-expression. Which
means, if you do the work to push past your comfort zone to do brave things,
you are less likely to judge others because you understand the courage it takes
to authentically be yourself. If you don't, it means that cringing at others can
become self-limiting; if we decide to shame other people, we create the same
limits of self-expression within ourselves. Shaming others prevents us from
our own expansion.

The lines we draw between acceptable and unacceptable forms of expression in others, the things we cringe at, are indicators of our own borders for
socially acceptable behavior—cringe is subjective. You are not the dictator of
what is and isn't cringey. Something that is horrendous to you, is delightful
to another! I always think of a quote from Dita Von Teese: "You can be the
juiciest peach in the world and there will still be someone who doesn't like

peaches." The reasons people do and do not like things, including your form of self-expression, have little to do with you.

Of course, we are going to experience inner resistance and that wriggly toe-curling cringe when we see someone express themselves if we have learned that this is "too much" or have been shamed for expressing ourselves. Cringe visits us all and it is not a bad thing. I believe there are two ways we can respond to witnessing someone crossing these inner borders of ours: we can either allow the cringey behavior to repulse us, contract our growth, and further solidify our ego position as "better than" the person we are cringing at; or, we can decide to observe it and allow the behavior to create an opening inside us, one of curiosity, expansion, and inspiration. A space where we can be in awe of this person, allowing ourselves to wonder, *What would my life look like if I were to follow my curiosity and be myself, the way this person does?*

Your expansion lies behind the cringe. All of it. All the cringey shit you avoid doing because you're afraid of other people mocking you in the same way you mock others in your head. That is where your growth begins. Starting your new business page. Wearing the clothes you want. Making choices that are "different" to what your peers are doing. Joining a club. Taking a new class. The way to make the world a safer place for you to express yourself is to "be" the safer world for others to express themselves. What might your life look like if you stopped cringing at yourself and dared to go for the things you want? If you allowed yourself to feel inspired by others who try really fucking hard, instead of cringing at them?

Life becomes so much more joyful when we allow people to be themselves, the compassion extends to ourselves too. No longer a critic, you suddenly feel the urge to participate. You get fed up of rubbing shoulders with the cynical judges and decide you'd rather be free, on the stage, frolicking around courageously with the people they call "cringe."

WHY DO WE CRINGE?

It's not "weak" to value the opinions of other people. Humans have a deep and natural desire to fit in and belong. Our brains are wired for survival, not joy.

If we were isolated from our tribe in ancient times, we would not survive. We would have starved or been mauled to death by a predator. Our brains have hardly evolved since then, and so we still instinctively avoid things that make us vulnerable to this feeling of social exile and tend to avoid "standing out" at all costs. In the words of Brené Brown, "*Fitting in* is about assessing a situation and becoming who you need to be to be accepted. *Belonging*, on the other hand, doesn't require us to change who we are; it requires us to be who we are."

DILUTING TO FIT IN

Every time I have tried to find belonging or "acceptance" from a group of people or a person, I have diluted myself. No longer potent, my "essence" gets lost in becoming whatever I need to "be" to be accepted by this group. Do you know this feeling? Maybe everyone drinks alcohol, so you do too. Maybe everyone judges a certain group of people, so you feel you must join in too. Any time you try to reclaim your personal "essence" within this group, community, or relationship, they do not like it. Maybe you decide to stop drinking and someone makes a weird remark. Maybe you decide to go and talk to someone from the group of people they judge. Maybe you decide to start reading self-help books in a group of people who laugh at spirituality. Our sense of belonging in these groups is dependent on following a certain set of limiting unspoken social rules. After unknowingly breaking these rules, we might realize that we do not actually "belong" to these people, that our place in the group is conditional on "fitting in," otherwise we risk exile. It is this fear of isolation that keeps us living small.

Every time I have been "exiled" from a group for disobeying the unspoken social rules, though initially traumatizing, it has actually set me free to discover my authentic fucking self. In this isolation, where I did not belong to anyone or anything, I could "belong" entirely to myself without compromising my personality. Because when we are a part of any "group" it can become harder to think for ourselves, when every decision we make is being filtered through the imagined ideas and judgments of the other people. *What will this person think if I wear this? What will this person say if I join a new club? Will this person stop being friends with me if I start to become successful?* But in my exile from these groups, the authenticity I had been bottling up inside me finally had the room and safety to ooze out of me.

I have had women isolate me from friendship groups in adulthood because I was "too intense." I was isolated in school by my friends when I started to "try harder" in lessons. Something as small as raising my hand in class would receive snickers of laughter, because I decided to start *trying!* I do not see myself as a victim, this is simply the structure of ancient tribal shame. We do not like it when people behave against the codes of conduct that validate our own behavior. I have been publicly shamed for my artwork, my expression, my writing, and my appearance, and each time I am shamed, punished, isolated, I am reminded of the truth that we actually "belong" nowhere, we can only belong to ourselves.

For a while we have to leave these groups, refuse to dilute ourselves, and become a tribe of *one.* When we can become comfortable with being alone, when we belong to ourselves, uncompromised, we take this sense of "belonging" everywhere with us. We feel no need to dilute ourselves and can feel at "home" everywhere we go. *Because home is in us.* It is this ability to be alone and to be authentically ourselves that will attract the right people *into* our orbit. But these new friendships, groups, relationships, or communities don't come right away. We don't leap from one shitty group straight into the perfect friendship group. Often, the people we want to be friends with don't know where to find us because we've been hiding behind an inauthentic mask. We will go deeper into how to handle the solitude of authenticity later. But for now, I want you to know that you are not alone if you have ever experienced being forced to be alone.

Social exclusion initially feels like a kick in the face from the people we thought loved us, we wonder what we "should" have done or who we "should" have been to make them accept us, but it soon becomes empowering when we realize that it's creating space for something new and delicious to enter our lives. When something does not want us back, it is

REFUSE TO DILUTE YOURSELF. STAY POTENT.

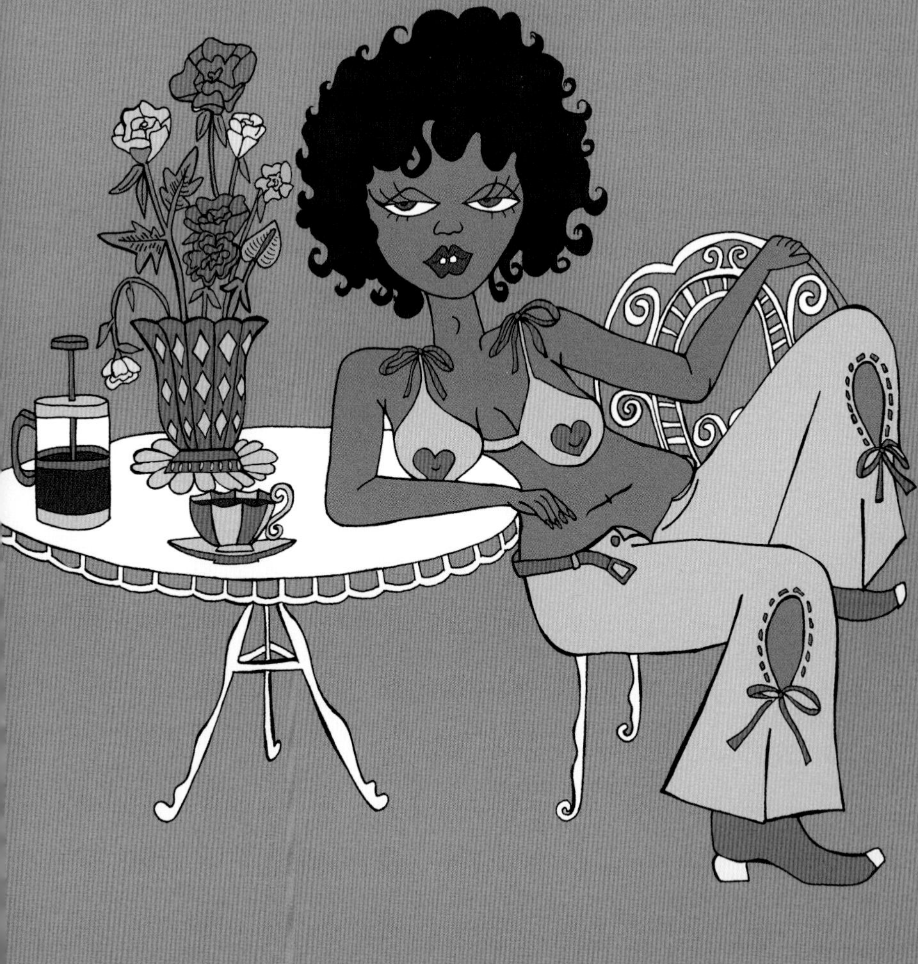

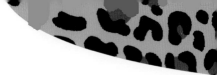

a blessing. We no longer have to waste time pursuing it and our energy gets redirected back to ourselves. We can expand into the space it left behind. We can finally grow into our authentic selves.

EMBRACING CRINGE IN THE FACE OF SHAME!

When we learn that it is not "cool" to be enthusiastic, that the people who are deemed coolest are the ones with an aloof detachment and disdain for self-expression, we enter this strange, growth-prohibiting competition in the race to be *the one who cares the least*, since this is what is now considered "cool." But what it actually is, is cowardice. It's safety. There is no risk in conforming. The people shouting, judging, and critiquing take no actual risk, in the way someone who bravely expresses themselves is taking a risk. In the words of Brené Brown, "There are a million cheap seats in the world today filled with people who will never be brave with their own lives, but will spend every ounce of energy they have hurling advice and judgment at those of us trying to dare greatly . . . If you're criticizing from a place where you're not also putting yourself on the line, I'm not interested in your feedback."

I want the very existence of this book not only to give license to people to feel that they are entitled to their small pleasures, their "cringey" self-expression, but also to give the small things that delight us a sense of legitimacy. We make things important by writing about them. By showcasing something, we enlarge it. We give it a place to shine. These "small" things that delight us are the anchors to joy in our own lives and the liberation from a cynical existence. The world fucking needs enthusiastic people!

We can often look at people who are joyful as though their optimism is ignorant, never stopping to consider how hard-earned it might be. What if their joy and expression is the part of them that *survived*? We tend to believe any display of real joy has been manufactured or is insincere, as though it cannot occur

naturally. What
is it about the releasing of
social norms we find acceptable if it is
induced through drink or drugs at a party, but
"cringey" if we are actively trying to change our outlook to be more positive? Why can't it be cool to *try*?!

    As a public person, I have had just about every aspect of my
personhood dissected, slandered, and ridiculed. But I don't believe
in the system of shaming. I want to continue to make the world safer for
people to express themselves. When we survive shame, and get to the other
side, a resilient confidence starts to emerge. It's the confidence of knowing
people have tried and failed to shrink you. The confidence of bouncing back
from shame is so powerful because you created it yourself and it is beyond
the realm of what can be destroyed. You can't touch confidence! You can't
touch joy! Remember what we said about invisible assets? They protect us
from shame too. We each have this untouchable place inside us. Remaining
in daily connection to it and strengthening it is what will protect us from having our sense of self destroyed by others. Find it, cherish it, and hold on to it.

FIGHTING THE CRINGE COUNCIL

The council of critical voices in our minds will often pipe up whenever we
try to express ourselves, trying to protect us from being hurt, but keeping us
small in the process. Here are two things they might say:

This is so silly and embarrassing.
We might be adults now, but that doesn't mean we should discard our sense
of play! For many of us, a sense of playfulness and ease isn't something we
have felt in our bodies since we were children, before our lives became filled
with responsibilities, perfectionism, and a heightened awareness of our appearance. While these ways of being are allies to our survival, they are the
enemies of playfulness and enemies of our joy. That voice in our heads that

tells us we are *silly for doing this* is just trying to protect us. But silly is beautiful, silly is playful, silly is where life happens! It's just being seen negatively by the serious perfectionist in us who has learned to view life as a stream of opportunities to prove our worth and win love from others.

I don't feel any better, "trying" is pointless.
No, it isn't. I promise you. You're used to things feeling good *immediately*, and having the shit feeling after. When something is actually good for us in the long term, we normally *dread* it before and feel the joy during the activity and after it. Being cringey and expressing the parts of ourselves we're used to hiding feels horrifying at first, but if we push through long enough we can feel the expansion it creates inside. The joy is longer lasting. We might not be able to get an immediate return on our investment or be able to calculate the changes in our lives from stopping to smell the roses, or smiling at a stranger, but we just have to trust that something beautiful is opening up within us, inching us closer to mental fucking FREEDOM!

EUUUGH, OH MY GOD, I'M SO CRINGEY AND DISGUSTING

Stomach-plunging, toe-curling embarrassment is normal. To be aware of how we are being perceived by others is frightening, and it often makes us want to shut ourselves off. The challenge here is to stay open, while the cringe is screaming in our heads. It is to keep doing what we're doing and allow the perception of cringe not to stop us. The best way to shake off a cringey moment is to not shake it off at all. Fucking own it. To decide, the moment we feel embarrassment, that we are not embarrassed. Insulate ourselves from the shame of others by repeating the affirmation, "I do not claim other people's embarrassment as my own." Don't delete the Instagram post because it didn't get enough likes. Don't remove the long, gushing caption and replace it with "photo dump." We come across these cringe barriers in our lives constantly and it is a great opportunity to build resilience. Slowly we realize it's absolutely absurd that everyone else *isn't* walking around passionately delighting in the miracle of life and the things they love.

BEING CRINGEY IS A PUBLIC SERVICE!

Still not convinced to come out of your cringe shell and dare to express yourself? Something I remind myself daily is that being cringey is a public service. Our authentic self-expression is a public service. Why? Everyone fucking benefits. When we lean into those impulses to laugh with reckless abandon, talk about our opinions honestly, launch a business, act on the impulse to turn our heads towards the sun, screw our faces up on the street because the song we're listening to is delighting us—we give all the people watching us a permission slip to be themselves too. Someone watching us thinks, *FUCK YEAH I want to be myself too!* Not only that, but the people who do cringe at us—the ones we're afraid will send our photos to their group chat, those who we're afraid will judge our work and write about it, family we fear will laugh about us over dinner—we have given *them* some fodder. What else would they have to talk about? They need SOMETHING. Something to boost their egos as they sit there telling themselves, *At least I'm not like that.* To them, we can say—YOU'RE WELCOME!

I like to view being cringey as "taking one for the team." Risking vulnerability for the sake of others' freedom. Risking vulnerability with the unwavering faith that this could allow someone else to become free too. Everyone wins when we express ourselves.

STOP JUDGING YOURSELF, STOP JUDGING OTHERS

Expressing ourselves is tough, but that's the point. We do something tough, and this forces us to realize that we're stronger than we thought. That even when people do make fun of us, we can start to see it for what it is—a reflection of their own limitations that were cruelly placed on them, the same way our limitations were placed on us. Someone once said to me that being a hater is like a "public admission of our own misery." It's hard to be mad at people who hate, once you realize that. Transmute their hate into love and send it back to them. They need it. Pray that they find happiness and for their every dream to be fulfilled. The peace this will bring you is immeasurable.

I have to check myself on my judgments of others all the time. They still fly into my head without my consent, and I'm often horrified by the weird and judgmental thoughts that can visit me. But they do not belong to me. They are not "me." They are clutter in my mind that I can ignore and choose not to endorse. We can all be better. Every one of us. The next time you feel yourself judging someone—or you feel the need to label something as cringey, ugly, too "trendy" or trying "too hard" —pause. Ask yourself what purpose does it serve your ego to feel superior to another person? We can utilize the cringe we feel as a portal to point our attention towardss the limiting shackles that exist within us, allowing them to dissolve. Allowing us to expand. To become free.

When people come for you—in school, at work, online—and you feel the walls of shame caving in; if you're tempted to succumb to this campaign of hatred, to change who you are, repeat these words out loud:

I refuse to be bullied out of being myself.

I refuse to be bullied out of my purpose.

I refuse to shrink in response to shame.

It's cool to try. It's cool to express ourselves. There are people who love the same things as you, and they cannot find you while you pretend to be something you're not. Let yourself be seen and just watch what fucking happens. Everything you want is on the other side of cringe.

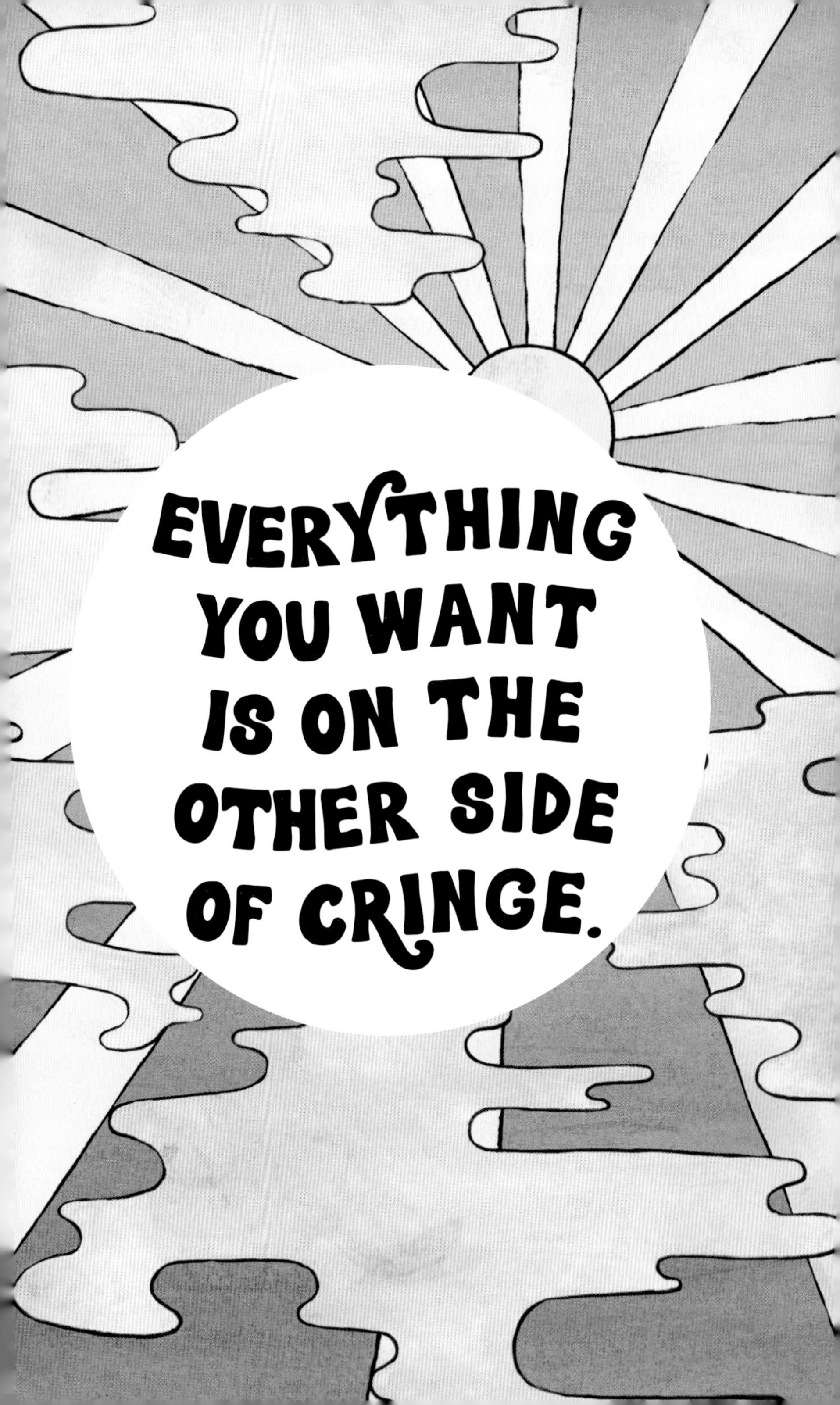
EVERYTHING
YOU WANT
IS ON THE
OTHER SIDE
OF CRINGE.

YOUR IDEAS ARE BEAUTIFUL

HONOR THEM WITH EXECUTION

Your ideas are beautiful, honor them with execution.
Your ideas are beautiful, honor them with execution.
Your ideas are beautiful, honor them with execution.
Your ideas are beautiful, honor them with execution.
Your ideas are beautiful, honor them with execution.
Your ideas are beautiful, honor them with execution.

Everything starts with an idea. This very book is the imperfect execution of an idea that existed as mere vapor in my mind! The imperfect translation of a swirling of thoughts that I typed out word by word, colors and concepts that I illustrated one by one, making them a physical reality. One sentence at a time. One chapter at a time. One illustration at a time. I almost talked myself out of it—why would anyone want to read my *silly little book* about joy? But then a second voice entered, the one that talks back to my fear. *Your ideas are beautiful, honor them with execution.* It became the affirmation I have repeated to myself throughout the process of writing this book. The courage that pulled me through to execution.

Expressing ourselves and our ideas feels less frightening and more EXCIT-ING when we realize that self-expression isn't supposed to be "perfect" or used as a vehicle to prove ourselves and earn love. The very act of expressing your-self has already fulfilled its purpose, because the point of self-expression is *to express! To contribute!* Expressing ourselves to receive praise, love, or attention can often set us up for misery. We end up suffocating the life and the joy out of the thing we're creating by placing the burden on it to bring us happiness, success, or love. Your self-expression does not need to be perfect. Self-expression is a vulnerable and generous act of contribution, courageously putting our thoughts out there to enter into conversation with the world.

Just like a great conversation, the best chats we have with people aren't perfectly rendered and polished, or a regurgitation of something we hear online, but those that allow us to see the world through the other person's eyes. Where you work through an idea together, trying to understand a subject deeper from both perspectives, and fleshing it out until we get closer towards something that feels like the "truth." By expressing ourselves imperfectly to another person, we open up to having our theories and beliefs changed and altered, examined, expanded. Perfectionism holds us back from the "messy" process that is necessary to EXPAND in life. The fearful voice of the perfectionist tells us that we need to have everything figured out, pretty and polished before sharing it with others—if at all. Our appetite for taking risks and being vulnerable shrinks when we listen to this fearful voice in our heads; it stops us from believing we can participate without "having all the answers." But guess what? No one fucking does. You just get better at articulating your inner world through practice. No one has ever found any answers without daring to be vulnerable and throwing themselves in to learn along the way. The mess is where you learn. Intentionally approaching life with a playful spirit and doing things even when I didn't feel "ready" changed everything for me. Because while I was holding back my ideas out of fear, there were people out there with half the skills but twice the courage to muck into action. These are the people who get shit done. These are the people who execute. There is no ceiling of limitation about what you can create in life, because everything is a learnable skill. You just have to put the reps in. Courage is all you need. Procrastinating can make you creatively constipated and block new ideas from coming through. Release yourself, get them out!

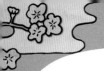

ALCHEMIZE YOUR PAIN

Self-expression is inherently imperfect because it is an attempt to translate how we *feel* on the inside with the use of *imperfect* tools—words, shapes, paints, instruments, our bodies, cameras. We express ourselves to *share* something we have found inside us. A feeling, an experience, a vision, an image. Great art and expression, in my opinion, is made when something gets as close as possible to articulating that feeling. This is why self-expression is the most sacred gift on the planet. This act of trying to translate ourselves not only helps us to sharpen our articulation of our inner worlds to others, but it helps us build our confidence as we switch from consumer, to creator. From being passive consumers of the world around us, to becoming active participants of expressing within them.

Your fear of other people's reactions should never stop you pouring yourself out. Sloppily. Messily. Beautifully. Wildly. It is the only way to improve, to get closer to what it is we want to express. We need to express ourselves to expand our thoughts beyond our limited minds. There's an expression I fucking love: *"All art is in conversation with each other."* Self-expression is so necessary to human life! Think of the songs that helped you through a breakup, the book that inspired you to quit a bad habit, the film that inspired you to pivot your career, the podcast that helped you through a dark time. Other people's courageous attempts at imperfect self-expression have been able to find their way to you, giving expression to something you also felt but didn't have the words for. Now imagine if the people who gave this gift of their art to you had decided to let fear win. To never publish that book. To never write down those lyrics that visited them on a walk. To not bring forth what was within them to inspire you. How drab our lives would all be! We need self-expression. It is the vibrant life force of human connection, the delicious thread that binds us all.

Consider this your permission slip: You are *allowed* to express yourself because you are a human being with a rich inner world that requires your voice, your words, and your body to articulate itself. *That* is your creative licence. No one else is capable of creating what you can create because your unique

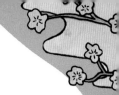

lens on the world, your unique set of experiences, has never existed before. Notice your surroundings, right now. You are the only person on the planet that currently has your exact viewpoint.

Your creative license is that you are HERE. You deserve to create, you deserve to express yourself because there is a whole world of intangible, universal feelings and concepts that we do not yet have the language for, that desire to be communicated through you, for someone to connect to something within themselves. The same way other people's art has done this for you.

Everything starts with a thought. Every building. Every book. Every album that has accompanied us in the beautiful and melancholic moments of our lives. It all starts with an idea. We just need to have the courage to flesh it out. That is what our bodies are here to do. To experience, express that experience, contribute, and learn. This is how we complete the cycle of expression, how we unblock ourselves, how we work towards making our "outside self" match the "inside self." How we get that delicious feeling of living in alignment with our thoughts, values, and feelings. Inspiration is good, but when we have been in a passive state of consuming the words and work of others for too long, we forget *we* can also create. Never forget that you are worthy of contributing.

No form of self-expression is, or ever will be, perfect. The whole *fun* of self-expression is in the process of teasing something out of yourself; a journey of getting closer and closer to the truth, each time an idea within you aches to lunge out and reveal itself. Why do you think so many books and songs exist on the same topics? We are all having our go at getting as razor-sharp close as possible to the truth. Human expression will always be imperfect, it is an articulation and translation of something you feel inside. Words are inherently limiting and always will be because we are using imperfect tools, words with definitions created by someone else, to communicate something that we *feel*.

MAKE YOUR OUTSIDES MATCH YOUR INSIDES

Every single action we take is building the reputation we have with ourselves. When we don't express what we want to say ("no, thank you"), when we break small promises to ourselves (snoozing the alarm every morning) or suppress our exciting creative ideas out of fear, we come to like ourselves less and less and our self-esteem starts to dwindle. When the "outside" doesn't match the inside, our lives can feel incongruent, and we start to build that inner resentment towards ourselves again. It fucking sucks. The good news is, it's simple to build back that trust. Taking small steps towards expressing ourselves is the antidote to this; by slowly ensuring that the outside matches the inside, we inch closer to the most magnetic and potent version of ourselves. We get closer to reaching our *potential*.

Every time we feel the urge to say or do something—voice an opinion, dance, sing, communicate our discomfort with something a person says to us, tell someone we love them—and we suppress that urge out of fear, our self-esteem takes a hit. It gets chipped away bit by bit. We slip back into that passive state. Every time we give in to our fear and don't share our work, or we give weight to the fearful voices in our heads that say we shouldn't say how we feel to a person because *it might make them leave us*, we learn slowly that we cannot count on ourselves. These small decisions build up, compounding over time, and it amounts to a deep feeling of passivity. This is exactly where I found myself after just one year of making small convenient choices to shrink myself in an attempt to avoid criticism from others. I became the most diluted version of myself possible. The message my subconscious received was that the design of my life was up for grabs, leaving others to be the architects of it. My life had taken the shape of my fears and the preferences of others. I started to resent myself—*How had everyone else become the central character in my existence?*

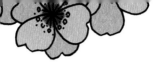

REFUSE TO DILUTE YOURSELF—STAY POTENT

The word "potent" is in "potential" for a fucking reason—we cannot dilute ourselves if we want to reach it. We need to stay potent. Making a habit of only expressing yourself in a way that you believe will be received "well" by everyone is a fast-track route to the most diluted and mediocre version of yourself. It's like adding more and more water to a cup of tea and wondering why you can't taste the flavor. You lost your fucking essence!

When we stay potent, refusing to dilute, we become the most magnetic versions of ourselves. Staying potent is how we reach our potential. The desire you have to create the life you want and express yourself must be bigger than your desire for it to be received *well*. It must overpower that fear of criticism. It is the only way we can build a life that feels authentically ours, with courageous self-expression that pulls us all the way through from our big and beautiful ideas, to execution.

You were built for bigger things. Small doesn't suit you.

EVERYONE STARTS OUT SHIT

We get better at expressing ourselves by pushing through the growing pains. It's very easy to express ourselves when we receive praise. Can we still trust that this is the right thing to do without it? When we share a concept with someone and they don't understand it yet? We need to trust that this is the only way we can get better at making our inner worlds into outer realities.

Successful comedians practice at small shows to refine their material before they do big tours for Netflix specials. Authors send their books around to editors and go through multiple drafts before publishing the finished version. It's such a vulnerable and challenging thing to express ourselves, because we're daring to expose a new, uncovered version of ourselves to the light. But in the words of Julia Cameron, *"All too often, it is audacity and not talent that moves an artist to center stage."* Having audacity in your vision, relentlessly trying to find better ways to express yourself, is how the outer and inner worlds will start to become more and more deliciously aligned. Embarrassment is just the cost you pay to becoming fucking excellent at something.

Elizabeth Gilbert, author of *Eat Pray Love*, says that in order to complete any journey we have to see "fear," the voice in our heads, as an annoying passenger that we have to take with us on a road trip. But we cannot, under any circumstances, allow it to stop us from going on the journey altogether. It sits in the passenger seat screaming the whole time, nagging, telling us we don't know what we're doing, that we might as well give up because other people have done this before. But if we wait for the fear to go, we never begin the journey. We will never be "ready" since we can never get rid of the fear. It's coming with us! Remember, the key ingredient is courage. We have to dare to express our vibrant thoughts, feelings, and ideas—EVEN when our fear tells us they aren't "good enough." We can inch closer towards our untapped potential.

YOU HAVE A CRUSH ON YOUR DREAMS, *RIGHT?*

When you think about them, you light up from the inside. They give you a little skip in your step. You gaze into the distance and your eyes sparkle at the thought of them. Flirt *back* with your dreams—they are flirting with you, so why don't you make a move on them? You can't stop thinking about them. Before bed. On your way to work. They fill the gaps of your day as you wonder about the delicious life they could give you. What are you waiting for? You know what moves you need to make. Start the researching, follow the Google tabs you still have open about classes, watch the YouTube tutorials, book the flight, listen to the podcast episodes. Tease your dreams out of you and entertain them as often as possible. Action them. Talk to people about them. Take one small step. Otherwise, your dreams may eventually leave you to find someone that wants to take them out on a proper date, someone who's all action.

Are your ideas going to change the world sitting in your drafts? Will your ideas get any better without feedback or review? Will the people you know you were meant to be surrounded by be able to find you if you're hiding in this watery, diluted version of who you are? When we hold out forever until we have got something *just right* before sharing it, we find that day never comes and we never share it at all, which is what our fear wanted in the first place. To avoid exposure. To avoid being seen. We make small tweaks, we edit things here and there, but we're still no further than the idea stage. It is because we are delaying vulnerability. It is because we are obeying the voice of fear.

You are not that fucking voice, but it will never fucking leave you. *You have to do it, even though you are afraid.*

Dare to express yourself.

Your ideas are fucking beautiful, honor them with execution.

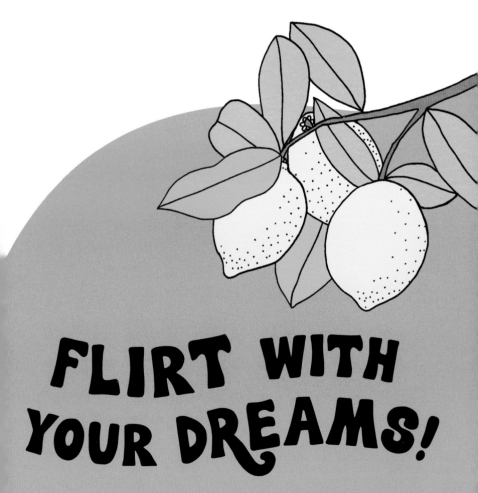

FLIRT WITH YOUR DREAMS!

I FUCKING LOVE PEOPLE.

I fucking love people. Tiny moments of human connection have saved my life. There's something so warm and connective about kindness from strangers that touches us in ways online connections cannot, no matter how much we have delegated our social lives to the internet.

Studies have found that casual and in-person human interaction, even with strangers, significantly contributes towards our longevity. But human interaction is becoming far rarer and ever more avoidable, particularly in cities where so many services have been replaced by a computer or delivery service. Even small human interactions, like asking the barista what the name of the song is they're playing, can be skipped over with the ability to Shazam it with our phones before we order our coffee. Next-day delivery means we can order a pair of garden shears, avoiding knocking on our neighbor's door to borrow some. Fuck, we don't even have to cook! We can spend more time at home working and hustling and order straight to our doors. Smooth, easy, quick, and efficient. This should be a good thing, right? FaceTime replaces a hang out with our bestie because it saves the commute. We do the same with our meetings, with dating. We remove the awkwardness of having to interact with people, prioritizing comfort and time. Humans will always choose the path of least resistance and almost everything in our lives is becoming as frictionless and convenient as possible. While many of these developments have been amazing in improving accessibility for many, I often wonder: is there a hidden cost to all these efficient choices?

I recently left my phone at home and walked to get a Chinese at my local takeaway instead of ordering in. I haven't done this in over ten years. I stood under the bright strip lighting in the waiting area with the smell of prawn crackers filling my nostrils, exchanging small talk with the other people who were also waiting. Everyone was wrapped up warm; the woman standing next to me was in her slippers and fluffy robe. The experience felt like a novelty that reminded me of my childhood. Of walking down to the Chinese on Saturdays with my dad and sneaking an oily chip out of the bag on the way home. I held the door open for a family, and each one of them thanked me on their way out, smiling at me with their bags of food. Through these brief interactions, the kindling was lit and that little bolt of warmth shot straight into my heart. I felt it melting the walls of separation between me and the world, having spent the day working at home. I got the bus home and a young couple sat in front of me smiling, with their heads resting on each other. I too sat smiling as I thought to myself, *Fuck. These are the mundane interactions that save people's lives. This is why we leave the house.* And sometimes, when we're in a pit of depression or the seasons' shifts are hitting us hard, leaving the house is an accomplishment all of its own.

These are the small moments that save people from loneliness. These moments have saved *my* life. It sounds wild to even be writing that. The kindness in the eyes of strangers that pulls us out of our own lives, even for a second, can remind us that the world's a bigger place than just our worries and stress. These strangers have no context of who we are, or the storm our minds are raging against us.

THE NEW CONTACTLESS WORLD

We are missing out on so much LIFE, on all that real and warm connection we need to survive. We are replacing it with the cold efficiency of contactless, quick, and smooth interactions. We are having to fight upstream against so much technology now because it erodes the human connections we used to get effortlessly. We used to have so much more contact, even exchanging cash with hands at the checkout every day. Now we use self-service, or tap with our contactless payments. Our existences themselves have become contactless. Efficiency has removed that warm romance and awkwardness of having to interact with human beings.

Of course, these advances were made to make our lives easier. But we have to ask, why do we need such contactless lives? If we're being encouraged to do things quicker so that we have more "time," what is it that we're doing with this free time? Are we using it to live more and be present, or are we using it to work and spend more time on our phones? Are we any happier? Or would the stress we feel about having to interact with people be conquered by having no choice but to face it? What if the automation of everything is making us less tolerant, resilient, and happy? We believe that we are gaining so much more time, money, and resources by creating an increasingly fast-paced society, by skipping the bumpy awkward parts of life. Meanwhile the cost and effect on our mental health of being "disconnected" is tallying up in the background. The value that we gain from interacting with human beings cannot be measured in money and tangible assets. We do not have a measure for the feelings, the sensations, the nontangible energies that sustain life. But they *are* felt in the heart. And they do matter to the quality of our lives.

DISCONNECTED

Now that we are able to interact with one another online without having to face the consequences, a strange duality is developing in people, emboldening them to behave in ways they would never dare to in person, for better or worse. It might be easier to face rejection by boldly asking someone on a date via sliding into their DMs, but it is also easier to let our ego run rampant and say horrific things about others without consequences. This disconnect is impacting our ability to engage with people offline too. By only seeing the things we already agree with, brought to us by the algorithm, we start to see our view as "right" and are shocked and appalled when something contradicts this. We are becoming less able to handle life and the multitude of contradictions it contains.

In addition, there are few consequences for the way we behave online. In fact, most of the behavior we see online would never occur in person. Online human interactions are pumped full of dopamine, but often devoid of the transformative warmth we experience by talking with someone in person. In her book *The Empathy Effect*, Helen Riess shares interviews with internet trolls, which she describes as shocking because they "don't tend to view their victims as real people." Empathy is reduced when we do not see someone as a person, but instead as an avatar. Now that more of our lives are lived online, we feel the disconnect even further as we have started to value our actions online as more important and having more weight than those in the real world. People are more concerned with their online "public representative" than their actual behavior.

The icky thing about doing "good" online is that it is so hard to quantify the motive behind an action, when all of it happens in the public sphere and is inherently performative. I fear we're entering a landscape where we can loudly profess online that we co-sign the latest trendy think-piece from our sofa while also harassing someone we don't know to "speak out" on the matter. Not once considering the real-life anxiety and fear we are causing another human by messaging them—all in the name of "justice." But really, we're just trying to assuage our guilt. We saw something horrible, we didn't want to feel bad, so we passed it onto someone else. I have been this person. A person in a chain reaction of triggered people, triggering other people. A lot of this is from a place of fear—we are more afraid of being seen as "bad" as opposed to being driven by a desire to do something good and impactful in the world. If "positive change" was our genuine motive, then the act should be carried out with compassion instead of moral superiority. Sharing the latest infographic about a crisis, getting our ego stroked by other people who praise us for being on the "right side of history," allows us to move on with our day and feel like we're good people and shame others for not following our example in the process. Meanwhile, in the real world, we're too afraid to get up and offer our seat to someone on a bus, hold a door open, or make small talk because we have lost our sense of social exchange and responsibility by delegating all our interactions to social media. We can come to think it's too "small" a gesture to matter. We can come to think that kindness, unwitnessed, offline, is a waste of time. The "pics or it didn't happen" mentality that social media brings out in us can contaminate every area of our lives. If no one sees the nice thing I did, *does it even matter?* But if we don't have patience to be kind to others in our daily lives while trying to make a difference in the world, then it's not about making a difference in the world, it's just another addition to the curation of our public image, controlling how we wish to be perceived. It's fucking hollow.

We're getting used to having everything effortlessly and without discomfort, which doesn't create the traits we desire for our future society, of patience, gratitude, and kindness. It breeds the opposite. Higher expectations, lower tolerance for discomfort and an entitlement to have things immediately. Our brains are wired to choose the path of least resistance, and if we keep choosing it, it is going to stray us further and further from ourselves as we default our choices out of immediate gratification and not what is best for ourselves and others.

The little things cannot be underestimated. The small acts of kindness, gestures, smiles, favors we do for people and that people do for us, are what build trust in others and ourselves, too. These interactions help us see ourselves in relation to the world around us, instead of closed in on our social media profiles, zoomed into the narrow view of our phones. We can do better, we can be better, and we must never forget in this fast-paced, smooth, and efficient world how important basic human kindness is to the people we interact with in our daily lives, as well as online.

THE COURAGE TO BE KIND

Have you ever wanted to offer help to someone, but didn't feel confident enough to leap in? Confidence doesn't just impact our ability to live beautiful lives for ourselves, it allows us to help others. But remember what we said about confidence? It's not born, it is BUILT. It takes courage! We may feel we don't have the confidence to interact with others, but interacting with others *helps* us to *build* that confidence. When we feel needed, when we feel important, when we contribute to the world around us, it actually boosts our self-esteem. We feel like we matter. No act of kindness is too small. It is never wasted.

I fear that as well as losing focus on the small and beautiful moments of our lives, we're also losing our ability to value the small but impactful acts of being kind and generous to strangers. Acting as though we have no responsibility to each other, metaphorically letting the door swing in people's faces behind us. The effect the internet is having on us means we crave instant gratification and quick rewards. It can be very easy to neglect small moments of compassion and responsibility towards strangers offline and discount them as unrewarding, settling instead for the instantly ego-gratifying work of displaying our "morals" online. If we want to detox from the quick rush of dopamine we get from likes and attention, we have to get used to not receiving rewards straight away, or perhaps ever, for acts of kindness. We may never see the impact of our kindness, we just have to trust that it's helping someone. We must learn to become satisfied with receiving nothing but that little bolt of warmth and connection.

LEAVE THE HOUSE!

Leaving home is one of the most basic needs for me, right up there with drinking water and getting enough sleep. Sometimes we just need to remember that the world exists outside of our heads! Even if we just go for a walk and smile at the person we see every day walking their dog. Do the same with the cashier and barista, flight attendants and bus drivers. Whoever we interact with on a daily basis, especially if it's transactional, we should make it our mission to infuse the interaction with as much gratitude as possible. Human connection cannot become a lost art, we desperately need to save it.

The world is less scary the more we interact with it. I never feel both more scared and more alive than when I take a little leap of courage and do something kind for a stranger. Paying for someone's snack or coffee in the queue. Helping someone with their luggage. Holding a door open. Reaching my hand out, expressing a compliment, and feeling part of something bigger. Feeling responsible towards people and helping in the smallest ways possible has unintentionally been one of the biggest confidence boosters for me. It makes me excited to leave the house. To experience the delight of human connection! Doing something kind starts a little chain of positive events that open up for you (and for the other person) during the day. They might feel energized to help someone else, too!

There are so many reasons to hate the world, but my god there are so many to fall in love with it. While writing this book, I was on a flight back from Vienna. I was seated right at the front of the plane, but my suitcase was placed right at the back. When it came time to land, I was prepared to wait for everyone to leave so that I could retrieve my pink suitcase. Instead, something beautiful happened. A passenger at the back of the plane passed it over his shoulder to the person in front of him, and the entire plane of passengers passed my suitcase over their heads to the front of the plane for me to leave. Even the flight crew were shocked. Everyone was smiling. Everyone cheered and laughed. It wasn't about me. It was the feeling of everyone working together. It was a big, fat, juicy moment of human connection and awe.

I have a million of these stories, some smaller, some bigger. But when we experience these moments, big or small, it reminds us that our lives don't belong to just us. That we can choose to be responsible for one another in the smallest, non-obligatory ways. If we want to live in a kinder world, we must *be* the kinder world we want to see. The "world" isn't some vague concept. The "world" is just *people*. And you are "people"!

You are a stranger who thousands of people will interact with in this lifetime. You have the power to leave the world a better place. Kindness is contagious. You can be the reason someone goes home smiling today, sighing in relief that the world isn't so bad after all.

I have witnessed the contagion of kindness so many times. I watched a woman in a café compliment a barista's outfit and he smiled his arse off about it! When he served me my coffee, he blurted out that he was "OBSESSED" with my outfit, wearing a massive grin on his face. It was not a good outfit. I was in a fucking tracksuit. It was clear that he simply had to unleash the

excitement he felt inside from being complimented and needed to get it off his chest.

A lot of the time we keep our heads down, not wanting to intrude on one another's lives, assuming everyone wants to be left alone. A lot of the time, this *can* be true, and of course we should be careful to respect other people's boundaries. But sometimes when you feel some kindness inside you that needs to be expressed, it can be *exactly* what the person needed to hear. The person whose dress you muster the courage to compliment may have spent half an hour at home debating whether to wear it or not because they were afraid of drawing attention. Now they feel fucking incredible and affirmed in their choice. They walk away with a skip in their step and feel empowered enough to compliment someone else's outfit later that day. How beautiful?! Kindness is contagious!

Sometimes, being intruded on in a beautiful and kind way is one of the best things to happen to us. It is like a little wink from the universe. I cannot imagine how beautiful the world would be if we each embraced compassion as a personal responsibility, ensuring that we take care of ourselves well enough so that compassion always feels like an option. That is a world I want to see. So that is the world I must be.

BE THE SIGN FOR SOMEONE

Sometimes we don't know why we need to express something kind, or creative, but we feel an inner urge—and we must act on it. Sometimes someone is literally looking for a reason to live. Someone is looking for a sign to leave their job. Someone is looking for a reason to feel good. *And we get to give it to them.* With a smile. With a compliment. By paying for their coffee. That person might have been asking the universe for a sign to keep going.

The trouble is, we never know who needs it. So we should be generous with our compassion to everyone. That does not mean we allow people to mistreat us, or take advantage. We can be open to the world while still having boundaries! Remember what we said about those gut feelings? Listen to them, always! But when we offer kindness in the world, we set an example that it is okay to involve ourselves with strangers to help one another, that we are all responsible for one another.

WHEN FEAR STOPS US HELPING

There are moments when reaching out and offering help feels scary, because it means we draw attention to ourselves. Even offering a seat on public transport or shouting to someone they dropped something. When you write it down, it sounds ridiculous that an act of kindness would take so much courage. But it does take confidence to reach out because it's so fucking vulnerable! I don't believe we're doomed, I don't believe we don't "want" to be kind. I believe we just haven't witnessed this generous way of being with strangers and that we don't get enough practice. I'm certain there are people rolling their eyes at this right now, people who cannot fathom not being able to interact with humans in this way. But it's real and it can be paralyzing for some people. We just need a little bit of courage.

Human interaction and social connection help us live longer. We don't need to have an enormous friendship group to live forever, we just need to start small. Start to infuse the interactions we already have with just a single degree more presence and we will start to feel happier. Why? Because when we connect with people on this fleeting level, we feel a part of something bigger. That our actions have an impact.

Do something small and beautiful and kind and don't tell anyone about it.

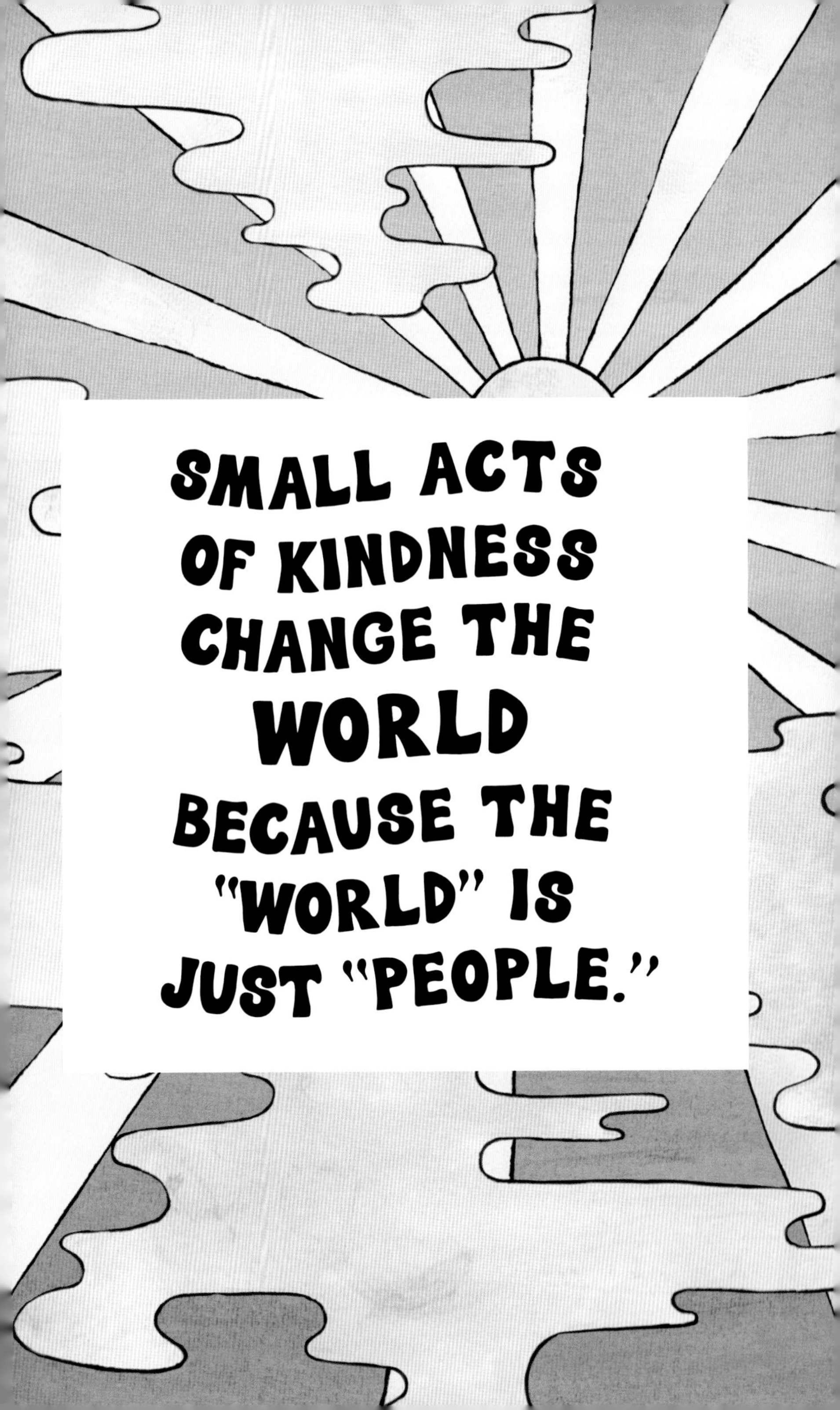
SMALL ACTS OF KINDNESS CHANGE THE WORLD BECAUSE THE "WORLD" IS JUST "PEOPLE."

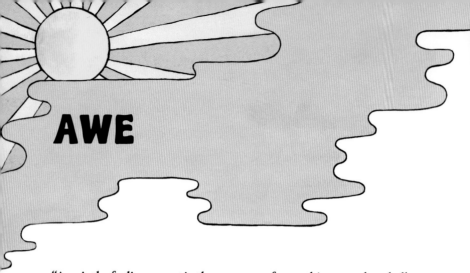

AWE

"Awe is the feeling we get in the presence of something vast that challenges
our understanding of the world."
—Dacher Keltner

What was the last thing you felt in awe of? The sky? Your lover? A gig? Your
pet? Awe is such a beautiful emotion. I am often moved to tears and overwhelmed by how in love with life I am. All I need to do is look for a reason—
and I can find it. I would have never dared to publish those sentences years
ago. Too gushy! Too vulnerable! Too earnest! But life is too short to pretend
you aren't in awe of something.

When we think of "awe" we often imagine something large, like seeing a
skyscraper or a shooting star for the first time, or witnessing childbirth. But
we can feel it in the small moments in life too. I experienced awe the first
time I witnessed a burning hot pink sunrise slashed across scattered clouds
in Tokyo, when I learned that some flowers close their petals at night, when
I danced so hard that I could no longer *think*, listened to a piece of music so
intently that it lit up every cell of my body, walked through a busy city and
felt part of something bigger, looked into the eyes of someone I love knowing what they're thinking. These moments may seem small, insignificant,
and without a common thread, but they do have something in common—
CONNECTION. They help us connect to something bigger than ourselves,
briefly escaping the "self" in our heads and reminding us that we occupy only
a sliver of this earth.

This connection to feeling intensely *alive* can be found in human connection, nature, art, music, and the beauty of our insignificance. It is so simple. It almost feels illegal because it costs nothing. Sometimes, to pull myself out of a slump, all I am required to do is leave my home. The world around us is littered with reminders that forever does not exist, that now is all there is, that our worries aren't all that important. That beauty exists in abundance all around us. That a new life is always possible. That we are not trapped in someone's else's script. That we can be the director of our existence. That no matter where we are right now, there is joy if we look for it. That there is always a reason to keep living.

THE MAGICAL VANISHING OF THE SELF

You've likely heard the word "ego" used as an insult before, but everyone has an ego. The ego is our sense of "self." It is our identity. The story we have about who we are. It is through this lens of our identity that we view and interact with everything in our lives. Neuroscientists have located the "ego" in the brain, in the default mode network we mentioned earlier. This is the area where the "self" lives. Dacher Keltner's research has proved that this part of the brain shows reduced activity in moments of awe. They allow us to expand our consciousness to something beyond our "self" and feel connection to something bigger than our ego-centered existence.

This is the exact thing that happens in our brains on psychedelic drugs. The "feeling at one with the universe" that you hear people say after their drug-induced high is largely due to the decreased activity in the "self" region of the brain. The "self" literally fucking vanishes, the veil lifts, and we feel at one with everything. Something inside us steps aside and it clears the way for connection to occur.

How. Wild. Is. That.

Dacher Keltner explains that one of the portals to experiencing this emotion of awe is through "collective effervescence." Isn't that the most beautiful fucking phrase you've ever heard? Collective effervescence is the feeling of energy when people are engaged in a shared purpose or experience—people feel it at church, in a packed cinema, a football stadium, a yoga class, or dancing in a crowd. A recent study found that at classical music concerts, audience members' heartbeats start to synchronize. But as we are increasingly attending concerts and filming through our screens, that fuzzy, collective effervescence has been fragmented into individual experiences. This has severed us from that delicious wave of human connection. We literally get cut off from the "vibe," which prevents us from experiencing as much awe as we should.

Awe is in the small moments of life that are so beautiful they break us out of our routine and leave us feeling connected to everything in a way that transcends language. Call it wonder. Call it awe. Call it sacred. Whatever you want. That warm, hair-raising, spine-tingling, fuzzy, chill-inducing feeling in our bodies in the "presence of something vast" is an emotion that brings us into the moment. Since the beauty of the thing we're appreciating commands our total focus on it, we forget our life stories and anxieties. For a moment, we are just blissfully *here*. Experiencing awe reminds each of us of our place in the world, but more significantly, it reminds us how insignificant we are. Awe makes our problems in life seem smaller. In the sunlight that reflects on the ripples of the ocean, in hearing a transcendent piece of music, we are able to not just understand, but viscerally FEEL that we are a mere and insignificant speck, contributing to the web of connection in the vastness of human life.

It turns out that in order to expand, we must realize how tiny we are. Keltner's findings prove that awe dramatically reduces stress, makes us feel a greater connection to the world around us, increases generosity, builds a sense of responsibility for others, and relaxes our nervous system. Meaning that awe—when integrated into our lives—has the power to heal us. It doesn't sound like a typical kind of path, to humble yourself to a mere speck, but the more we get out of our heads, the more we are anchored in the present moment, and the more we can feel connected to the joy inside us, underneath life's shame, distractions, and fear. Awe is a tool we can use to tap into that reservoir of joy inside ourselves.

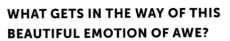

WHAT GETS IN THE WAY OF THIS BEAUTIFUL EMOTION OF AWE?

Fear. Distraction. Thoughts. Simply not paying attention. These are all things that make it harder to access awe. However, just like gratitude, awe can be the way out. We can stop waiting for it and start to seek it.

We start off with a great ability to experience awe as children, asking questions, acting intuitively and curiously. We have no sense that something is embarrassing until we are taught it. Our curiosity becomes suppressed by cultural norms. Our lives become moulded by the environment we grow up in. We need to become self-reliant, make money, manage our time, be great at our jobs, a good partner, mom, friend. Somewhere along the way we lose our connection to curiosity. Our vibrant inner world depreciates, not in one fell swoop, but with each small decision that suppresses our curious nature. The idea of awe starts to feel "silly" when you have work, chores, bills, and responsibilities.

But there is no dress rehearsal for life, there is only "now." Life does not begin one day in the future. It is now. And one day we will draw our last breath and the privilege of having a body to live it will be gone. Bronnie Ware published a book, *The Top Five Regrets of the Dying*, recounting her years in palliative care. The top five regrets of patients were:

1. I wish I'd had the courage to live a life true to myself, not the life others expected of me.
2. I wish I hadn't worked so hard.
3. I wish I'd had the courage to express my feelings.
4. I wish I had stayed in touch with my friends.
5. I wish I had let myself be happier.

Bronnie expanded on the last regret by adding, "This is a surprisingly common one ... They had stayed stuck in old patterns and habits. The so-called 'comfort' of familiarity overflowed into their emotions, as well as their physical lives. Fear of change had them pretending to others, and to their selves, that they were content. When deep within, they longed to laugh properly and have silliness in their life again."

People who are dying wish they had allowed more silliness into their lives. I would say that is a pretty urgent fucking call to embrace your playful, awe-inspired, curious inner child. At any time, death could come. We do not know when, yet most of us live with this false certainty that tomorrow is promised. Life is just a succession of small moments. If we do not stop to appreciate them, they will pass us by. There is magic in everything, we just need to find it in something "bigger" than us.

Whenever I forget this, I find something in the present that can act as an anchor into the "now." The breeze rustling through a tree's leaves. The craftsmanship of a spider's web. The way the things left on my desk have been scattered, almost like a shrine to the past, showing each of my habits and movements. The creases around the eyes of the person I love which offer a glimpse into the lines that will one day permanently form on their face. There is magic in absolutely everything around us. It's ironic that in order to expand, beyond our problems, beyond the turmoil of our minds, we must find something which reminds us of how small we are. How bittersweet a truth it is to acknowledge in these glimpses how transient life is and how many of the details we miss in the busyness of looking forwards, always on to the next thing.

THE SPARK THAT NEVER LEFT YOU

When you feel like it's been a while since the magical veil of awe has visited you and life has been feeling flat, remember it is still there. It might just be harder to locate. We never lose that inner wonder, awe, and curiosity, not even through trauma or the numerous responsibilities we have in adult life. The path back to feeling hope is through seeking it out.

We tell ourselves that we cannot afford to stop and notice these moments. *Who has the time?* But the opposite is true. We can't afford to let these moments pass us. We often look around at everything we've built and wonder why it is still not enough. Why is it *never* enough? Because the beauty is in the journey and the journey is what we're skipping over.

Most of our lives are spent hustling and slogging along to achieve one milestone after the other—school, a degree, a job, marriage—making choices to fast-track us into a life we're told will bring us happiness "when we finally achieve this big thing." And yet, immediately after achieving the milestone, we feel empty. The insatiable void inside us, of course, fucking wants something else. This cycle is known as the "hedonic treadmill." The cost of not ever slowing down to enjoy our lives—IS our lives. We will never get those minutes, days, months, or years back. Time is a nonrenewable resource. Under capitalism, we're made to feel that any time spent "not working" or being productive feels like time "wasted." We cannot fathom that there is room for both, a dance between playing our roles and also relishing, time for both expansion and rest.

LIFE IS YOUR LOVER AND SHE JUST WANTS YOUR ATTENTION

I like to imagine that life is a patient lover, just waiting for us to pay attention to her. If we're not careful and we continue to pursue more and more external pleasures, the joy that lies in the small details of life and the spaces we inhabit daily goes unnoticed. We become numbed. The new freckle on our partner's face. The entire meal we ate without paying attention to the taste in our mouths. The flowers planted outside our neighbor's house. The bird song in the morning that sounds like nature's flirting with us.

If we do not pay attention to these small ways that our lover—"life"—is trying to connect with us, we sour the relationship. We lose our relationship with joy and awe the same way a lot of happy couples lose their connection with each other—by slowly choosing the easy option of comfort and turning away from connection. This is how our relationship with life becomes toxic. John Gottman, a relationship expert, can predict divorce with 93.6 percent accuracy. He developed something called the "bird theory" to test if a relationship is doomed to fail or last. The test is to see how your partner reacts when you point out a bird to them and say, "Look at that bird!" How do they respond? "Where?" or "Wow it's so beautiful." If the partner is disinterested or doesn't engage with what you're saying, or dismisses you, it's a sign that the connection in the relationship isn't healthy, because they dismissed what Gottman calls a "bid for connection." This applies to any attempt that you make towards your partner or your friend. You could ask them for help. You could sit next to them on the sofa. Do they turn away, by getting out their phone? Or do they turn towards you and lean in for a cuddle? Whether or not someone chooses to "turn away" or "turn towards" you during a bid for connection, Gottman argues, determines the quality of the relationship.

I believe his theory can be applied to our connection with ourselves and our relationship with life. The more we turn away from our curiosity, the more we reject the "bids for connection" that life extends us in the beauty of small moments where she tries to reach out and connect—when a strip of sun lands on your face in the morning or a bird perches on your window—those are the moments when life is making its move on you. That is life flirting with us! When we ignore these bids for connection and pull out our phone or glaze over them, it's like receiving a handmade gift and tossing it away in favor of a shinier pleasure we get instant gratification from. We keep skipping over life's bids for connection to prioritize entertaining dopamine-hit distractions, like going back to the toxic ex who gives you a good shag but leaves you feeling immediately shit afterwards. It may be fun and thrilling in the moment, but it's not a sustainable relationship and it's damaging for your long-term health and happiness.

When we neglect to pay attention to life, our connection to joy becomes a distant memory, the same way a couple in the chaos of filing for a divorce might look back at the joy on their faces in wedding photos, wondering how they got here. This joy we once felt becomes a state of being we cannot relate to. The more we continue prioritizing jobs that don't fulfil us, opening up apps out of habit, chasing pleasure instead of sitting in silence and delighting ourselves with what's around us, never letting our minds settle for long enough to notice life's signs, her bids for connection, never taking steps towards the life we truly want to inhabit—the more we ask ourselves, *Why am I so unhappy with life?* The disconnection happens slowly. Incrementally. Which means it can be recovered slowly and incrementally too.

Most of us have a toxic relationship with life which we run or numb out from. Filling the gap between us with "stuff" to avoid feeling her. Scrolling.

THE COST OF NOT
EVER SLOWING DOWN
TO ENJOY OUR LIVES
- IS OUR LIVES.

WE WILL NEVER
GET THOSE MINUTES,
DAYS, MONTHS
OR YEARS BACK.

Booze. Shopping. But all she wants to do is hold our hand and ground us, reminding us that there is joy to be experienced. We can repair this relationship with life by asking ourselves at any moment, *Does this decision I'm making feel like I'm turning away from myself or towards myself?* Turning towards life could look like leaving your phone at home before you go for a walk to see what life has to say to you. It could be following your curiosity, when you feel intrigued by a question, a color, an observation. This entire book is the result of me following my curiosity about the architecture in Japan. I looked up at the sky and observed that all of the balconies in the buildings were facing away from the sun. I started to wonder how much happier the residents would be if they could wake up to sunshine beaming through their windows. It led to a journaling session where I decided I always wanted to "turn towards the sun" and listed the things that make me happy in life—and this became "*ways that I like to live deliciously.*" You have no idea where looking up and out can take you. Look up. Look out. Turn towards life. She has answers for you, but you will need to slow down and pay attention to her first.

P.S.

If a song could hold your hand and gently remind you to slow down, it would be "Vienna" by Billy Joel. The lyrics heal a part of my urgent, perfectionist mind that wants to keep chasing and achieving. This song feels like a love letter from life asking me to slow down and love her. Give it a listen. I hope it feels like a hug.

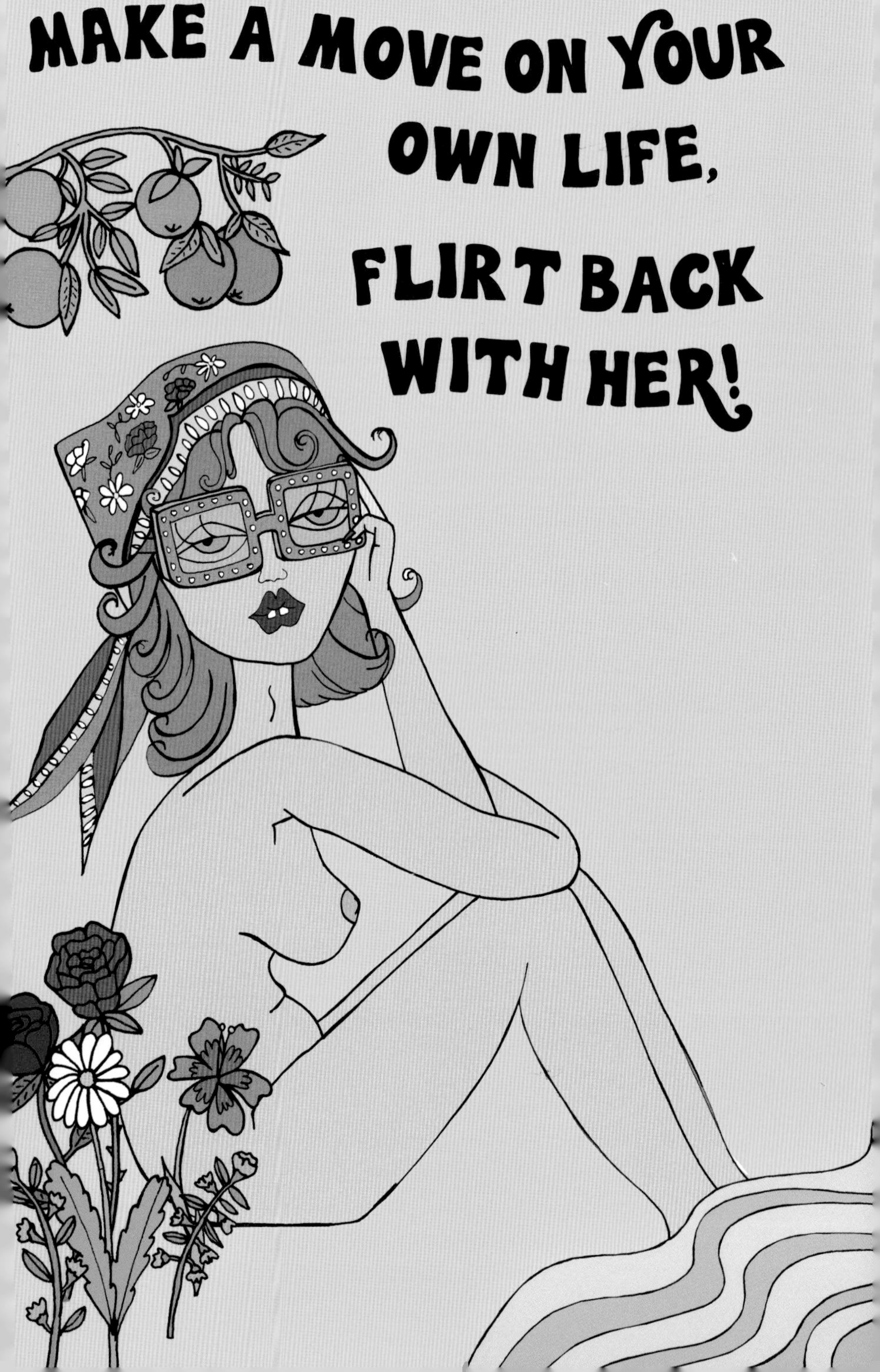
MAKE A MOVE ON YOUR
OWN LIFE,
FLIRT BACK
WITH HER!

HOW TO PAY ATTENTION TO LIFE, YOUR LOVER

The beauty in the simple things goes unnoticed when we do not slow down. Beauty and abundance are all around us. But they are playing hide-and-seek. We have to slow down and pay attention to find them. This is a little practice we can do to reconnect with life, to turn towards her and open up the possibility of seeking and finding joy again.

By either locating something of beauty—noticing the way someone you love has done their hair—or *creating* something of beauty—intentionally hanging art in our homes—we feel less helpless and become empowered as active seekers of joy and beauty, instead of passively waiting for it to visit us.

Just a few seconds spent intentionally observing beauty grounds us in the present, we get to relax our nervous systems and create breaks from performing our roles. Doesn't a few seconds of appreciating random intervals of the day seem manageable?

I'm going to talk you through what this "slowing down" process looks like for me. This is a very basic example of mindfulness and something I use daily.

So. Let's set the scene.

• You're living your life, minding your own business

Let's say you're brushing your teeth. Your mind starts to wander, you are now performing the action without much thought. It's almost like it's happening without you there.

● **Enter . . . the incessant inner monologue of your mind**

This is so boring. When was the last time I flossed? A week ago? That's embarrassing. Oh god, imagine if someone knew I hadn't flossed. I wonder if that's a turnoff in dating? Oh, I should check my dating app requests later. I'm single. Ugh. God. I hate being single. I just want someone to love me. But who could love me? I don't even floss my teeth. I'm pathetic.

● **You've gone on autopilot**

Suddenly, what was a simple activity has become a trigger for unpleasant thoughts to start popping into your head. Because the action you are doing is on autopilot and does not require your focus, your focus drifted to your thoughts. But remember, these are not the thoughts that you have consciously chosen. The thoughts that we hear in our brains are not "who we are." They are the internal chatter of the default mode network we discussed earlier. It could torment you about anything.

Something about your body.

Something about a person you're jealous of.

An insecurity.

Anger at someone who's eating loudly next to you.

A mean and judgmental thought about a person's outfit.

An expired argument with someone you knew from high school that your mind has decided to bring up . . . again.

● **Stop and notice it.**

When the thought arises in your head, simply notice it.

Catch it.

Watch it.

Observe it.

This might sound obvious, but most of us do not stop to notice our thoughts, we allow ourselves to be dictated by them and *become* them. It is hard to notice that the voice is not who we are, because it's happening in our heads. But our thoughts are merely tools. So as soon as a thought comes up, notice that it's *happening to you* as soon as possible, before the next thoughts follow on the same negative frequency and drag you down with them. Did you notice how quickly it happened?! Michael Singer describes this process as creating a duality. When you notice and observe a thought, you create a duality. A subject-object relationship, between you and your thoughts. You are able to observe them—as you would observe a flower on a walk—as an object, outside of *you*. This separation is crucial before the next step.

● **Great news, you are no longer in the fog!**
You are no longer inside the thought, like being in a patch of fog with your vision blurred. You are looking *at* the thought. You are looking at the fog. You can now start to feel the space between you and the thought, you can realize that you never were the fog, but that you are the sky that contains it. Once you have noticed it, you want to sustain this distance between you and the fog—the thought—as gently as possible. You want to maintain that gap.

● **Locate something of beauty**
Hook yourself into this state by finding an anchor. Observe your surroundings. Find something beautiful in your environment. Something that pleases you.
     Find something silly. Find something delightful. *Find it and use it as your anchor!* The mind can only hold one thought at a time. By shifting your focus onto something beautiful, you replace the negative thought with a new one. An object of beauty, the scent of your coffee, a person, a puppy, the feeling of fabric against your skin, the breeze in the curtains, a toothpaste stain, someone browsing the supermarket aisles, the items on your desk scattered messily. Absolutely anything.
     The world is the best art gallery. Observe it as though it is a piece of art, or as if the world in front of you is a scene in a movie. Find something you didn't notice about it before. If you can't see the beauty in something, it's because you're not paying attention. Look deeper. It's going to feel so fucking hard at first, especially if you're in a shit place. But it's possible. I have once found inner peace by staring at the back of a man's head while descending the esca-

lator on the Tokyo metro. I thought about how the spiral pattern in his shaved head replicated patterns we see in nature. My mind started to wander into these pleasant thoughts as I had delighted myself with a reminder of how connected we all are. I couldn't help but smile. My attention had successfully shifted from the narrow focus of my negative thoughts and onto the world in front of me, reminding me of my insignificant place in it and quietening the anxious thoughts of my mind.

Found something? Okay. Now that you have found your anchor...

• Take a deep, belly breath
After you have found something to focus your attention on, take a deep breath. This will bring you gently into the present and keep you here for longer. This will hold the distance between you and your sticky, unpleasant thoughts so that they do not suck you in and drag you down. Try to observe the beautiful thing you have chosen for as long as you need to feel something shift slightly inside you.

If you feel like you want to further pull yourself out of the spiral, you can take it a step further.

• Create a moment of beauty
Now you need to take some inspired *action* to enhance your experience, bringing you further out of the stinky poo of your brain. Open your phone and play some music. If you can't trust yourself not to get distracted on your phone, play a CD or vinyl.

Dance to it. Get into your body. Open the curtains if they're not open. Look out of the window. Put your shoes on and go for a short walk. If you're already walking when the unpleasant thought strikes, choose to stand still or sit on a bench.

Make your screensaver into something that brings you joy, so that you can view it in these moments. Repeat an affirmation to yourself that you prepared for these moments, something like: "NOT TODAY!" Smile. Laugh at yourself

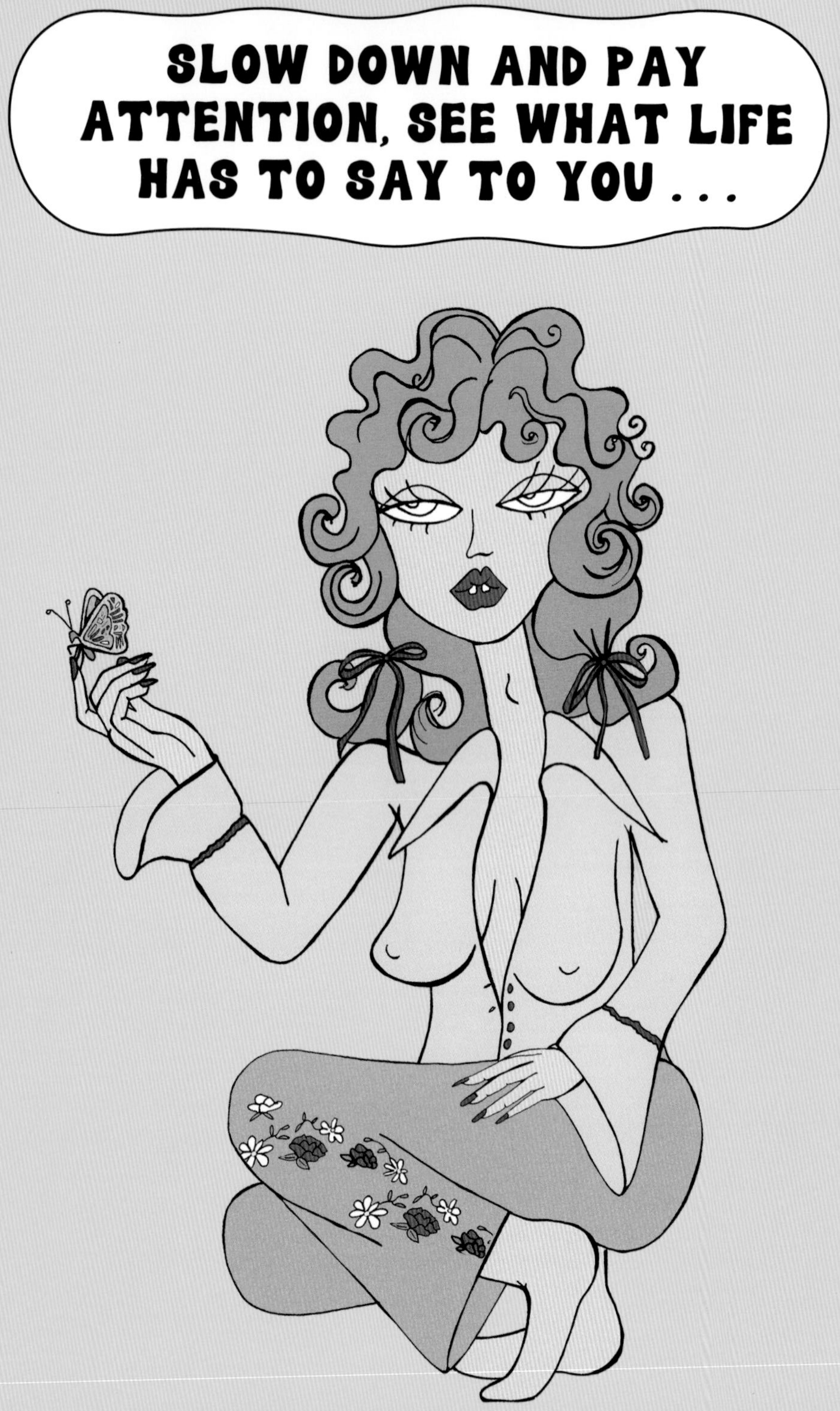
SLOW DOWN AND PAY ATTENTION, SEE WHAT LIFE HAS TO SAY TO YOU . . .

GET OFF YOUR FUCKING PHONE, I LOVE YOU.

and the hilarity of your punishing mind. Call a friend. Pay attention to the activity you're doing. You need to *do* absolutely anything. By taking action that gets us out of our heads, we rewire the familiar path in our brains of "rumination" and begin to forge a new one. The agency this brings us is remarkable. What I've discovered is the thoughts that come before an unhealthy habit I'm trying to kick, scrolling or picking my skin, were the catalyst for those habits in the first place. Kicking those habits starts with noticing those thoughts.

This is how we become the master of our thoughts, instead of our thoughts becoming the master of us. There are anchors in our environment absolutely everywhere. It doesn't mean the anxious thoughts we were having disappear, but they now exist without the energizing, multiplying power of our attention making them worse.

This entire process feels a lot like a computer coming back "online" after it has been on autopilot. I like to think of these small things of beauty in my life as "anchors" because the term conjures a sense of "grounding" for me when my head feels cluttered with the fearful voice that kicks its way back in to irritate me.

DELICIOUS DISRUPTIONS

For the moments that bring us into a state of awe involuntarily, I use the term "delicious disruptions." Like a little wink from the universe. I can be sitting in the most beautiful park and in my head be having an argument with an old mate I haven't seen for literally years, and a butterfly will land next to me, taking me out of my stream of thoughts, forcing me to erupt into laughter at the ridiculousness of my own mind. The ability to laugh at yourself is one of the best skills you can possibly develop towards living a joyful life. We can use the world as our anchor and the delicious disruptions as our own accountability partners in helping us to stay present.

A bird.

A plane in the sky.

A flower growing out of the cracks in the pavement.

A joyful child.

A crack of sunlight shining on the floor.

A song you love on the radio.

Anything that feels like a *wink*.

We can use delicious disruptions for anything. Even helping us to reframe seemingly negative events too. Is it an inconvenience, or a delicious disruption? We never know if an event is protecting us from something. It might at first seem forced, silly even, to be in a traffic jam and late for work and tell ourselves, "this is a delicious disruption." But the effect that framing inconveniences and things out of my control has had on my mental health has been immeasurable. As with anything, it is not what is happening, but the story we tell ourselves about it that leaves the impression. If we cannot control the thing from happening, why not change how we view it? The ego loves to have reasons to feel as though bad things are happening to "me" all the time, but the more we practice reframing situations that are actually just neutral, the more power we have over our own lives. What is this trying to teach me? Perhaps patience. Perhaps, this is an opportunity to think. What if the annoying couple hogging the pavement in front of me is an opportunity to slow my pace? Perhaps I am in this traffic jam because it is preventing me from a dangerous incident. Perhaps this delicious disruption of a child jumping into puddles in their wellies, of the delay of a train, is providing us the perfect gap of awe to stop and turn towards life, towards ourselves, that we have been craving all week.

The next time something minor happens outside your preferences, I want you to try telling yourself that this is a delicious disruption, even that you are grateful for it happening. Not because it's what you wanted to happen, but because it happened and there is literally nothing you can fucking do about it. You restore your control and sense of agency when you tell yourself that you can be glad it happened, instead of being a victim to life and the things that drag us around. You enter another level altogether when you can be grateful for the disruption.

The process of stopping in the middle of what we're doing to look around and remind ourselves of our environment:

- Creates new pathways in our brain to stop negative thinking as default.
- Reminds us that we have the power to choose differently and say "NO" to the tormenting voice in our minds.
- Restores our sense of control over our lives and boosts self-esteem.
- Brings us back into the present moment.
- Reduces self-consciousness by looking out at the expansive world around us, instead of focusing on the narrow "self."
- Relaxes our nervous systems from "fight or flight" into the "rest and digest" mode, required for healing to begin in our bodies.

If we practice this daily, for a few seconds or a couple of minutes, we start to notice that our minds look for awe and the beauty in little things without us even commanding them to. It starts to feel like bliss on demand. We wonder how we went so long without noticing that there's a bush of flowers in our neighbor's window box. Or the beautiful way our barista does their makeup every day. The tattoos someone has. We wonder how many other details about our lives and the world we were missing. But the joy was there the whole time. The awe was there the whole time. We just have to train ourselves to notice it.

STOP AND SMELL THE ROSES

How can we give ourselves *permission* to relish and enjoy the experience of being alive, instead of waiting to have bodies "perfect" enough that "deserve" to relish in life? How do we move away from the peripheries of our existence, paralyzed by the fear of jumping into play, experience life, and look silly? How do women relish and enjoy our lives *now*?

The ridiculous simplicity isn't lost on me, that the key to accessing more joy for most women is simply becoming wise to the proper use of our bodies—that earth-shattering realization of *Holy shit, my body is here to help me experience LIFE? Not to be skinny and pretty?!* We are severed from our connection to our bodies so much, forgetting that they love us, that they are here to help us live, experience, with all our senses to enjoy it. The decoration of those bodies is supposed to be the fun part, not the stressful part.

Among my life's greatest pleasures are summer and sex, but they are also the times when I am most likely to objectify myself, preparing for them like my life depends on it. The sun being out should mean we jump for joy, but it's often underpinned with a dread of exposing our bodies, the parts we normally hide under clothing, the blemishes on our skin or the cellulite. It's the same with sex. *Which positions make my stomach look good? How can I lose weight in seven days? How can I impress them? What noises will they like?* The inherent pleasure and joy in these activities can get sucked out when we view them instead as obstacles we must tackle and "get through" due to the pressure we feel to be pretty and perfect, instead of being present, experiencing what it means to be

ALIVE in these moments. The pressure might even prevent us from enjoying the experience altogether.

Do you understand how fucking absurd this is? It is heartbreaking to consider that most of the events I have canceled or not been present for can be boiled down to the fact that I did not think I looked good enough to attend them. How cruel that our minds convince us that we are not good looking enough to live our own fucking lives. We deserve to feel, we deserve to RELISH, that is what our bodies were made for. Refuse to gatekeep yourself from your own life. Life is about *living*. That is what we are here to do as human *beings*. Experience everything that life has to offer. Taste things. Smell things. Experience the art of other human *beings* in books, at galleries, in music, consume their expression and interpretation of this thing we all experience called "life" and to also create our own. Life is for experiencing the full range of human emotions—grief, awe, sadness, heartbreak, joy, euphoria, boredom.

But the more we become aware of how much we are objectifying ourselves, the less power it has over us. We can choose to take the other path. To stop giving that habit of self-surveillance strength. One beauty distraction resisted at a time.

Prioritizing our *experience* of the world, as opposed to how we *look* while experiencing it, is the way out of our collective self-obsession and self-surveillance. Big or small, find out what makes you feel alive and lose yourself in it as much as possible. You deserve to live just as much as the "thinner" or "prettier" version of you that you have been using to punish yourself with in your head. The version of you that you are now gets to LIVE. NOW. I am not implying this is easy, but that you are worth taking the first step. No matter how "small" the step is. *You* determine when you start living, not the mean council of voices in your head. You can expel them and replace them by living and loving every second you have on this planet. Opposing them with one intentional action at a time in the pursuit of your fucking joy.

Most of us live our lives the way we eat a meal, only becoming aware that we should relish and savor it when it comes down to our last bite. Our lives are incredibly short. We cannot wait until we feel deserving or "worthy enough" to prioritize our pleasure and experience of the world. We must do things to

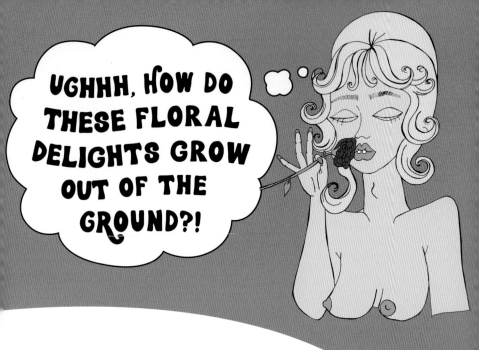

intentionally *inspire* that feeling of joy within ourselves. Life is bittersweet. We're here for a short while.
What do you want to do?

I want you to live this life so fully, to be so intensely fucking
HERE for all of it, so that you can rest satiated, full, exhausted, not
from a life lived in chasing, pleasing, and perfecting, but exhausted from
having lived so fully, with a satisfied smile on your face and messy fucking
hair, like life *itself* was the best shag of your life. Seizing this one precious gift
you were given, *to be alive*. Living deliciously is about asking ourselves, how
can we make the present moment more joyful? And soon, it will not just be
a habit, but a way of life.

What scents do you love?
What things do you like to look at?
What do you like the taste of?
What sensations feel good on your body?
What music or noises do you love the sound of?

Build a life around these things. They will help you get into your body.
Don't forget to honor yourself by changing with them as they evolve.
To allow your joy to be the architect of your life.

SMELL

1. Inhale the scent of a fresh loaf of bread! Stop to inhale when you walk past a bakery. Put the fucking croissant up to your NOSTRILS.

2. Quite literally, stop and smell the roses. It feels like a crime to walk past a rose bush and not stop to plunge my face into its center, letting out an exhale so audible it sounds orgasmic. I was once sat on a bench enjoying the morning sun when a woman zoomed past me on her run, smiling at me on the way. I then watched as she stopped, out of breath, to pick a sprig of lavender from a bush. She rubbed it between her fingers and continued on her run with her fingers stapled to her nose, her eyes rolling back. DELICIOUS!

3. Smell the coffee brewing as it wafts over to you, or as the freshly blitzed beans grind in a coffee shop. Don't worry about looking "silly." Doing this in public has actually pushed me through so much of my

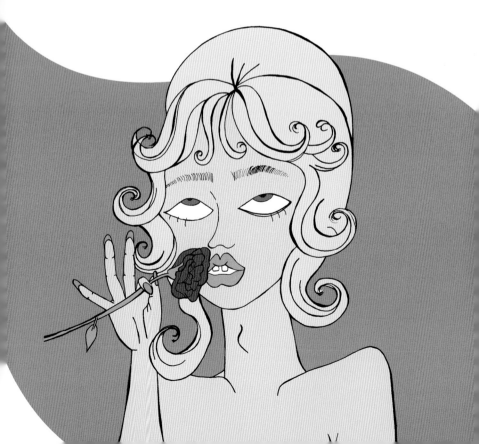

social anxiety, to relish in whatever I want, whenever I want. Smell the rim of your cup before you drink it seductively each morning. ORGASMIC!

4. Cook with fresh ingredients rather than buying something ready-made, even if you start with only one night a week. Do not view this as a chore, but a *luxury* for your hands and tastebuds. A treat. You deserve to spend the time creating something to feed the body keeping you alive. The smell will fill your kitchen with warmth and delight!

5. Go to an incense store and spend as long as you desire sniffing the different scents. Pick out your favorite and buy a pack. Take it home, light it in your room, and open a window. Create a little altar for gazing into the sky, put on a great fucking album, and watch the tendrils of smoke fade out, changing their shape every second.

6. When you're near the ocean, inhale it ALL. Breathe in the delightful fresh scent of salty air and the wide ocean crashing on the shore.

7. SMELL A PERSON YOU LOVE! Your baby's head, your partner's head, your friend's new perfume when you hug. Relish in it all.

TOUCH

1. Sex is an experience, not a performance. A lot of us grow to believe it's a performance through porn. But it's a way to feel pleasure. One way to feel more embodied during sex is to consider whether a position even *feels* good, or if you're doing it because you think you "should." Would you rather dry hump and make out for hours than have penetrative sex because you connect better this way? Suggest it! Remember, it's about your *experience*, not the story you tell your friends, or doing something you don't want to do because you think it will make them happy. If it's not a fuck yes, it's a "NO."

2. When you buy a bouquet of flowers, or one is gifted to you, spend some time noticing the details, touch the petals, the stems. Can you notice anything interesting about the flowers you didn't notice before? The tiny hairs? The shapes? Some flowers have hairs on the

backs of their petals—can you feel them? Can you now touch the tip of your nose, your cheek, and feel how, you too have hairs on your skin?

3. Wear comfortable clothes. Wear the outfit that doesn't suck the shit out of your stomach and isn't going to ruin your night. That doesn't mean to say you need to live in your comfies if you feel it dampens your self-expression, but, if you can, invest the time in curating a wardrobe that both expresses your personal style and makes your body feel amazing. Sell stuff that doesn't fit or hurts you when you wear it. We have internalized the message that "beauty is pain," but your body is here to EXPERIENCE, remember!

4. For some reason, a croissant will always taste better out of a crumpled paper bag than it will served on a plate. A pizza will always feel more romantic when you eat it out of the box. A drink always tastes better in a cold glass. Noodles taste better with chopsticks. Make a meal out of how you experience your food. Whatever that feels like for you!

5. Wash your bedsheets, even if you are tired. The small act of preparing fresh sheets for yourself and getting into bed is a reminder that you deserve to be taken care of.

6. Make your bed, it sends the message to your brain that you are organized, that you can take great care of yourself. It's also what's called a "keystone habit," which means it helps us make healthier choices throughout the day. Remember that Future You needs to be cared for after a long day and doesn't want to get into a bed that hasn't been made with care for tonight's sleep.

HEAR

1. Almost every single moment of my life is improved by soundtracking it with music. A walk through a chaotic night in Soho can be turned into a scene from a movie by listening to Pink Floyd. Create the score

of your life! Soundtrack it all. Create a playlist for yourself for every emotional occasion. The memories you hold for specific moments in your life can unlock beautiful nostalgia. Playlists for trips, events, will always make me feel warm and fuzzy inside.

2. CHANGE YOUR MORNING ALARM, FOR THE LOVE OF GOD! I hope you do not wake up to the sound of a horrendous phone alarm. It triggers so much anxiety in me to even hear it. I bought a real alarm clock a few years ago, and it's changed my life being able to wake up to the (fake) sound of birds chirping. The habit of being yanked out of my blissful subconscious dreamy resting state into a high-cortisol state of anxiety from the sound of a pounding alarm was horrendous for my mental health.

3. The sound of birds unlocks something in me. I didn't hear them for a while living in the middle of the city, and it wasn't until I heard them in a park one day that I realized how much they were missing from my life. I make visits to parks a regular activity now. Sometimes it sounds like the birds are flirting with me and my heart SWELLS! What sounds of nature delight you? Find them!

4. Relish in the sounds of the world around you. The clatter of cutlery in a restaurant. The sound of motorbikes whizzing past. The wind. People's conversations. If you pay attention, you will notice the sound of a hot sunny day in a city is different to a gloomy day. It just *sounds* hot. I CANNOT EXPLAIN IT BUT IT'S REAL! Listen to the sounds around you in moments of anxiety, or gaps between activities, instead of reaching for your phone. Try to find a sound your mind didn't pick up before. What can you hear in the layers of noise of the world?

5. Really listen when someone speaks to you. How do they sound? Can you focus entirely on them talking, without being distracted? Can you try to bring your attention back to them as much as possible?

TASTE

1. Eat fruit that you have to peel and pull apart with your fingers. Buy an orange or an enormous fucking grapefruit and peel it apart. Smell the zest as you tear the skin. Pull the segments out from their skins and look at the little transparent juice pockets. Feel them burst in your mouth. Burst them individually with your fingertips. Taste them. It is the most sensual experience ever. If you focus on nothing else but peeling, opening, smelling, and tasting a grapefruit, I genuinely believe it could induce a spiritual AWAKENING!

2. Take yourself the extra mile to go to your favorite food store, or your favorite restaurant. Is the pastry you want a farther walk? Go fucking get it for yourself like you would for the love of your LIFE. Something beautiful and new might happen on the walk, too! It's so good to change up our routes, just as we do with trying to change our habits. Walking different paths forces us to think consciously because we can't perform the route on autopilot.

3. Try something new. Get to know your local area more. Is there a new food place that's opened? Try somewhere you've never been because you've been waiting for someone to join you. Your life belongs to YOU! Your culinary experience should not shrink or bloom according to the schedules of other people, so when planets align and somewhere is exciting, affordable, accessible, and welcoming, embrace it.

4. Sit with the sensation of the food in your mouth, experience every mouthful fully. Do not wait until the end to realize it is almost over.

5. Do not give a shit about how you look while you eat. If your eyes need to roll back because that sumptuous, nutty, caramel, and chocolate dessert is causing an oral orgasm, ROLL THEM BACK! RELISH RELISH RELISH! Close your eyes if you want.

6. Eating is a great time to practice gratitude. I always think of something I'm grateful for before eating and if I'm at home I will say it out loud. It literally slows me down and forces me to be present before I dig in.

SEE

1. The lighting in your room can be so important. If you use overhead lighting in your bedroom, make sure the bulbs are at least a warm white, not a cold white. Or buy yourself a lamp with a cute shade that brings you joy instead. An entire room can be transformed in an instant with warm, cozy lighting. Overhead artificial lighting can make a room feel clinical and messes with the melatonin in your brain, making it harder to sleep.

2. Change your phone wallpaper to something inspiring, or fill your walls with art to ignite inspiration! The reason people don't stop going on about vision boards isn't because they're "magic" but because they reinforce an image of the life we want in our minds and every time we look at them, we are refocusing our attention towards our goals. Our minds remain open to the ways that life is trying to invite us to step forwards and take action.

3. Dress to delight the shit out of yourself! Simply changing the question from, "Is this enough?" every time you look in the mirror to "Do I feel delighted?" is game-changing. Because instead of making the world the judge of beauty, you are now making yourself the judge of beauty—and dressing like THAT. Or, sod beauty altogether and dress for comfort. Who cares what you look like? When we dress according to our own delight, whether people validate the outfit or not becomes irrelevant—it has our stamp of approval already.

4. Getting my nails done does something fucking WITCHY to my self-esteem. I am more expressive. I am more confident. Suddenly I can't stop talking with my hands. I look at my hands all day when I am writing on my laptop and the visual delight often makes me stop

to pause and appreciate them—whether it's extensions, a simple gel coat, or just filing them. There is a correlation between my self-esteem and my nails, and it is NOT superficial!

The practice of enhancing our lives through our senses in these small, sustainable ways reminds us that we are here to experience the world and all it has to offer, including other people. Engaging in our lives in this way reminds us that we are not objects, it is a small step out of the paralyzing state of self-objectification that we have learned. Often when we execute these little rituals, it is not just the thing we're doing that brings us joy, but the agency and self-esteem we derive from making a conscious choice to change our environment and take control. Sipping that coffee instead of gulping it down reminds us that *we* can control ourselves. Research even shows that moments like this, of appreciating beauty, actually relax our nervous systems and can bring our bodies into a state of healing. Neuroscientist and author Dr. Tara Swart suggests that this could be because in ancient times, if we had enough mental resources to stop and appreciate something beautiful like a flower, it must have meant that we were safe and not trying to outrun a predator. Appreciating beauty sends a signal to our bodies that we are safe and brings our nervous systems into a relaxed state where they can finally heal, instead of allocating all our resources to surviving in fight or flight. Through this process of appreciating beauty, we can go from merely surviving to thriving.

These small moments prove that we can be creators of our reality rather than victims of it. We slowly rewrite our story, one action at a time. It is a little window for us to peer into a different life that we could live for ourselves—one full of joy, connection to the world around us, awe, and gratitude. One where we rebuild our connection with life as we turn towards her, where we are not stuck and beholden to our default habits and programming or the expectations placed upon us by others.

Your body was born to RELISH in this unique experience of life. It's time to act like it.

SOLITUDE IS SACRED

If we want to experience joy, to understand our intuition, it is of great importance that we learn how to be comfortable with our solitude. It is only in solitude, when the thoughts and opinions of others part from our minds, that *our* truth and desires can burst into view like the sun through the clouds.

If we cannot push through the discomfort of solitude, we often find ourselves reaching back for the people and habits that aren't good for us. We always want to "fill" those gaps of silence instead of holding on to them and seeing what arises in this space. The ability to hold on, to continue to choose ourselves instead of things that harm us, is our "staying power." The longer we hold on, the bigger the gap becomes between our old lives and the people we are striving to be, and the more we start to call in and attract the things that are meant for this new version of us.

Most of us do not want to let go of relationships or attachments to things we know are bad for us, unless we know that there is something better waiting to catch us in its arms. But most of the time, life does not fucking work like that. It requires all our faith. We have to leap and trust that something else is better, without being able to see it. It sucks, but we don't leap out of one bad relationship and straight into an amazing one. There is a period of time when we need to belong to no one other than ourselves. To stop trying to attach ourselves to others and become what they want from us. If we have been seeking acceptance in others for a while and suppressing parts of ourselves to fit in, for a period of time we need to belong to ourselves. We need some time to recover all of the parts of ourselves we lost to the relationship, to the addiction, to the numbing, or the group of friends we have now outgrown. Those parts of ourselves that we suppressed beneath need space to grow. But they will not bloom and grow to their fullest capacity if we keep filling that space with more clutter, more people. There's no room for the shoots to burst out.

It is impossible for us to know who we are when we have a constant deluge of other people's thoughts, voices, and opinions in our minds. If we're healing from toxic relationships, our perception of reality has been skewed so much that it can require intense solitude to get back to our own thoughts. We need to see what visits us in the quiet. It is so incredibly beneficial to find and create gaps in our days to be alone, even if that's just in our own minds, so that we are able to check back in with our intuition, see how she's doing, and see whether or not we have gone down the wrong path. Every once in a while, we want to reach in and ask her, "*Is this what you really want?*" The answer you hear shouldn't be "*Yes, because it makes everyone else happy*" or "*No, because then my friends will laugh at me.*" It needs to sound like a "*fuck YES*" or a "*fuck NO.*" It needs to be a choice you would make regardless of anyone else's approval.

Though it may feel frightening, being alone allows us to get in touch with our authentic self behind the roles we play in our lives. Without the time alone, it can become difficult to know where the roles we play end and where "we" begin. In order to know ourselves, we must spend a lot of time alone, yet spending time alone for women is not only mentally but also physically frightening. As we discussed earlier, it is not just this internal idea that women need to "get over," but a real danger and threat that has instilled a fear of being unsafe in public when alone. With caregiving obligations and culturally enforced people-pleasing, articulating we need time alone can feel like telling someone we don't love them.

The reason solitude is so fucking powerful for women is because in this space—whether it's being single for the first time, being in a relationship and going on a trip without our partner, or going on a walk without our phone— we discover what we are capable of without distraction and other people's preferences filling in the blanks *for us*. In solitude we can finally hear what's *within us*, not outside us. We'll never know our potential if we always wait for permission from other people to tell us when to do something, where to go,

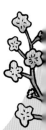

or who to be. Have you ever even tried doing something without asking for someone's opinion on the decision? Posted a picture without asking what someone thinks? Booked a trip? Chosen a film? Decided what to order on the menu? Decided what time you want to have breakfast instead of when everyone else eats? What works for YOU? I still often find myself having to resist polling every life choice with the people closest to me over WhatsApp. But every time I make a choice of my own without consulting someone's opinion, I feel more powerful and resilient. And if you're not in a position to make the big choices yourself, are there tiny decisions you can make that give you a sense of some control? This is how we stay POTENT. When we default our lives to the preferences of others, we never get to learn what it is that we actually want for ourselves or discover what we're capable of on our own.

How do *you* want to structure your life?

Unwavering faith and confidence in ourselves is built when we can become extremely comfortable with being alone and making decisions alone, because it forms this unbreakable trust in ourselves that we can take with us everywhere. This is why I love solo travel! There is no one to consult but myself. I am forced to trust my instincts when alone in a foreign country—where to eat or which direction to take on a walk. Making decisions for ourselves, alone, is the only way we can build a relationship with our intuition. It becomes our own internal compass. And guess what? If we make a "mistake" and choose the wrong thing, *we* get to learn from it. Through solving a problem, we discover we don't need saving. *We* can save ourselves! We need to learn things for ourselves, with first-hand experience, otherwise it does not get stored in our bodies as wisdom. We need to feel, discover, taste, and understand the texture of who we truly are so that we can bring this whole self to the encounters we have with people. Individuals meeting each other who can come to compromises, *without compromising themselves.*

Most of my relationships before I started this journey were like enmeshed melting pots, where I didn't know where the lines were between me and the other person. If we do not get clear on what it is that we want, if we do not know ourselves, then who we are will always be up for compromise and era-

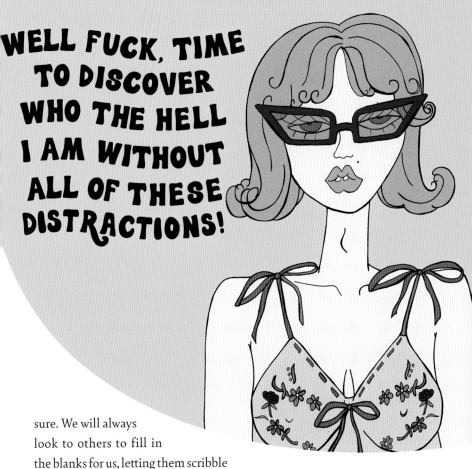

WELL FUCK, TIME TO DISCOVER WHO THE HELL I AM WITHOUT ALL OF THESE DISTRACTIONS!

sure. We will always look to others to fill in the blanks for us, letting them scribble on the dotted lines of our life's unanswered questions because we do not trust we can find the answers out for ourselves.

I had no clue if I was really shaving my body hair "for me" my whole life, until I binned my razors after a relationship and found I didn't pick them up again for years. I couldn't create an intentional relationship with sex until I embraced a long period of celibacy. I had to know, *was I bringing people home because I really wanted to, or out of habit?* I didn't know if I actually enjoyed alcohol until I stopped drinking. Turns out it was a habit of comfort because I wanted something to do with my hands at parties! When you stop or reduce your time engaging with certain things, you realize a lot of the time that they were the stabilizer wheels you no longer need and forgot to throw away.

It angers me that spending time alone has been so stigmatized and made dangerous for women because, if you can push through the fear, it is one of the most juicy, enriching, delicious experiences ever. It really is the difference between staying at home because our fear has told us to, and saying "fuck it" and going out spending the whole evening snogging someone sexy we met in the corner of a dimly-lit bar, or making a best friend in the bathroom. We increase the number of directions life can take us when *we* finally decide we are ready. Not when we feel ready, when we *decide* we *are* ready. When we make the first fucking move on our life and flirt back with it.

When I first chose to embrace solitude, I had many nights sobbing into my carpet clutching a glass of cornershop wine, wondering if anyone was ever going to love me and if this "growth journey" thing was even worth it. I thought self-care was pointless if no one was around to watch me do it. A lot of the time the fear we have around being alone can be put down to a desire to be witnessed, watched, experienced and to be felt, seen, and heard. Which is so fucking REAL. We feel that if we do not experience something in the presence of another, the joy or the act or the experience is wasted. But it could not be further from the truth. My life *began* when I decided not to sit around waiting to be invited to the banquet of life, and chose to roll up my sleeves and create my own fucking feast. No longer starving, I went from being a woman who constantly asked what she needed to become and what parts she should hide to be tolerated in the lives of others, to a woman who decided to make a delicious banquet out of her own life. With my own banquet, I could now be more generous. I was abundant, overflowing, no longer relying on other people's handouts of love and validation. I became the source of those things for myself and able to offer them to others too. This is what self-love is. It is loving yourself so much you never feel you have to settle for the scraps from others. If I had continued knocking on the doors of other people, hungry for their love and acceptance, I might never have looked within to discover that I was already in possession of all of the ingredients to live deliciously.

It is far lonelier to be in the presence of a person who doesn't see us in the way we deserve to be seen, for our full humanity, than it is to be physically alone. Being alone is the "break" we need from overstimulation and external opinions to be able to find out what it is we really want. Being alone is our reset. Being alone has nothing to do with isolation, or going off grid to find yourself, it is to retreat temporarily now and again within yourself so that you are able to discern more clearly the borders between you and other people. Once we begin to listen to ourselves we realize we do not need to "see things through" with people who treat us badly. We can recognize disrespect the moment it fucking happens. We develop the powerful skill of discernment. Other people's disrespect starts to become very loud when it contrasts so starkly with the trusting love we have created within ourselves, *for* ourselves. Accepting less than we deserve is no longer an option, but UNFATHOM-ABLE.

The relationship you build with yourself will affect every single other relationship you have in your life. Do you even know that a lot of the relationships in your life are a choice? That you do not have to maintain them out of obligation? Living a life of your design involves creating some space, carving out solitude and looking deep inside—but you can do it as slowly and gently as you like. There is no rush. Eventually, you will trust yourself implicitly. No more seeking confirmation on what you already know is right for you. The answers will not come from your partner, your friend, your therapist, an article, or this book, all others can do is give you the confidence to find *yours*. Or more accurately, give you the courage to act on the things that deep down, you already know.

The answer is in you. Do you have the courage to stop looking for signs? Can you act on what you *know*?

LOVING YOUR LIFE WHILE YOU HAVE ONE

Your body is a beautiful vessel that exists for your soul to experience life. It is a conduit, a gift, a medium for self-expression. Just as paintbrushes are tools for painting, our bodies are the mediums through which we express ourselves and experience life. Our bodies are not here to be desirable. They're here to help us express ourselves and live. The tricks our minds play on us, convincing us we are not good enough, are not *our* thoughts. They have been planted in us and it is our job to weed them out. No one else in the world can do this for us.

I always *knew* intellectually that people were worth more than their bodies. Yet this still didn't change how I *felt* about my body. It was not a powerful enough paradigm shift, to move the needle forwards in how I experienced my body in daily life. I "knew" women were worth more than their weight, *but still bought weighing scales in January.* I "knew" women should be able to relax without thinking about their appearance, *but still raised my chin when jolted into awareness that it had doubled with my posture.* I started to consider whether women were ever supposed to relax. Or would we always be taught to live exhaustedly, frantically, pleasing, and perfecting everything?

In the necessary feminist discourse about how "a woman is so much more than her body," I noticed that any counter-narrative to the beauty-obsessed one fixated heavily on a woman's career. Or it emphasized that women aren't just pretty, they're also moms, sisters, daughters. Although far better than how *pretty* we are, the focus of a woman's identity was still offset by what we could provide for others and how perfectly we could do it. None of this empowered me, none of this answered the question of *who am I when I'm not in relation to someone else?* Who are we behind all the roles we perform and the masks we wear? I started to think about how much our roles, no matter how fulfilling they are, can be made redundant if we change or the world around us changes. What if our partner leaves us, or we outgrow them? What happens when our children grow up? Or we lose our job? What if we're an athlete and we break our leg? Who *are* we then? Who are we behind these things?

All of these identity markers focused on accomplishing something, or doing something, or being somebody's *something*. A woman could only relieve herself from needing to be beautiful if she found and sought worth outside herself in another arena—such as her accomplishments, her earning ability or what a great partner, mother, or best friend she could be. It felt like we could never escape this trap of perfectionism, of needing to find a new "identity" when one dissolved or our priorities shifted in life. Would it ever be enough for us to just ... *be*?

None of the shifting identities I had adopted in my life tasted like freedom. Even being a "feminist" became a label that started to feel suffocating as I struggled to live up to every single one of feminism's values. I felt that there was something deeper still to what a "woman" is, and how even the idea of a "woman" was based on a set of beliefs and ideas made up, which women were socialized into adopting. "Caring" and "nurturing" are traits that many men are also capable of, it's just that we don't actively encourage these in them, we culturally accuse them of being "girly." What is a man? A woman? I found the definitions were limited by archaic, outdated stereotypes. When I peeled back the layers, I realized that all these labels meant absolutely nothing if they could all be stripped away in an instant to new information, to death, a change in beliefs, or to the uncontrollable, unpredictable nature of life.

So what is the thing that stays, when our roles expire? In the gap before we latch onto a new identity after the dissolving of another, who are we?

If I am not a body, but I *have* a body, then my body *exists* as a vessel to experience life, because my soul can't live without it.

Why am I punishing my body for the way it looks, when it was created to *experience*? My soul can't experience life without my body. She doesn't have arms. Or legs. Or fingertips. Or a clitoris. Or a tongue. She *needs* my body to live. I'm here to use this body to live the most delicious fucking life possible. To connect. To enjoy this planet. My soul doesn't *care* how my body looks! She just wants to go to a park and sit on a bench, the beach, savor every meal, walk the streets of a foreign city, smell the new air after disembarking a plane, feel the sun on her skin. The body was built for joy, pain, experiences, and sensation. The soul doesn't know the difference between a "good" body and a "bad" body when it's having an orgasm, or when it uses the tongue to taste food. This body is another creation of whatever energy it is that created all things, the higher organizing principle none of us can agree what to call. I am an expression of it. The same way my writing is an expression of me, the same way the orange is an expression of the tree, or the song of the bird. My body is a fucking gift I have been so ungrateful for, for so long. Your body is a gift to you, too.

Live as though the ghost of your future self is hovering above you, envious that you have a body to move, a voice to speak truth with, a mouth to taste food with, legs to dance with, a nose to smell it all. Imagine how frustrated she would be if she watched you punish your body, as you deem it not deserving enough for doing the thing it was supposed to help you do. Our bodies are conduits for our souls to experience the world. Cherishing them is a matter of urgency.

The thing inside us—our soul—is a wave, a temporary, unique, and brief expression of the wider ocean it rises from. A wave that can often forget it's connected to something bigger until we slow down to look around, watch, and observe the other waves crashing, remembering that our separateness from the world is an illusion, that we are all rising from the same ocean. We remember this connection in those delicious moments of awe.

When I forget I am not just an individual, but connected to something bigger, life can feel dull. It's in those small moments of connection—when I notice the soft hairs on the petals of flowers and delight in our similarities, when I watch a flock of seagulls turn their heads to face the morning sun in unison just as I do, when I witness strangers in love, when I look at the stars and realize how fucking tiny I am—the soul in me remembers that I am a wave, connected to the rest of that ocean. In these little winks from the universe are the bids for connection extended to me by life. As though life is constantly trying to remind me, *You are not alone, there are so many things to live for, you just need to seek them out.*

This is the reason some people have a creative idea that resonates with a huge number of people, because it came from "fishing" deep inside themselves, dipping into that bigger ocean that connects us all. It resonates with people because it comes from the collective pool we're all connected to. When I forget about this connection and I feel blocked up by the distractions of the mind, I start to judge others, I stop taking risks—I feel "off." Uncomfortable. Itchy. Irritated by people. I start to feel poorly. *Disconnected.* It is as though something within me is pushing me to get back to balance, to remember what matters. To remember that I am part of something bigger, that life is vibrant and there are reasons to live. What *is* this force, this part of us all that aches to bloom and expand? Our energy, our intuition, our soul? I do not know. Call it what you will. But I refuse to argue with her anymore. I know that she knows best. There is something inside us all aching to express itself, to use every opportunity for living as much as we can. Every time we complain about our bodies, our souls laugh, wishing we only knew how lucky we are to have one at all. We can find her within us, in the quiet. If you learn to listen to her, she will help you to truly live.

The soul just wants to *experience. Will you let her?* She wants to create through you, she wants you to use your hands, your tongue, your ears, your eyes—to create, dance, play, and experience the world. The soul doesn't care about the size of your thighs when you're at the beach, she just wants you to use them so she can walk herself into the sea and experience the sensation of the ocean on her skin, to taste the salty water on her lips. She wants to *remember* that connection to something bigger. Through music. Through dancing. Through kindness. She wants to experience the world. The soul is

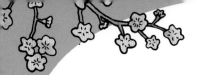

here to have a fucking good time. You are here to have a fucking good time! To feel the joy of being alive in a body with senses, to feel that connection to something bigger. That's what your body is for.

When you die, you will no longer be able to experience this physical world. The gift of your body will likely decompose, rot, give life to the ground around it. Your soul, your essence, *you* will no longer be able to sniff fresh pastries, no longer be able to travel and wander the streets of a foreign city, or hear the symphony of clashing and clattering of people's plates as they eat in outdoor restaurants. You will not be able to taste new food, or inhale the wafts of perfumed women on their way to a date as they strut confidently past you, you will not be able to use your fingers to feel the pulse of orgasmic pleasure, you won't be able to experience the satisfaction of a good night of sleep after a long day of work. When your time comes, I promise you that your soul won't punish your body for the way it looked, but mourn it for the things it allowed you to experience. You can choose, now, to embrace life as the luxury it is, while you have a body to live with.

When I think about my life from this perspective, I feel myself wanting to deeply love and look after myself. It charges me with the courage to talk more honestly, more vibrantly, to no longer dim that spark inside me I've been hiding from others, to live as vibrantly and compassionately as possible, talking to people the way I would if I had died and been sent back for one more day. *How can I be annoyed at minor inconveniences, when it's a blessing to just be here?!*

I want this feeling for everyone. The first moment I spoke "back" to the voice of fear in my head, I realized that my life belonged to me. I realized that we all have a choice, not just to ignore the voice in our heads, but to act against it and courageously create the life we want to live, one step at a time. We are not held captive by our thoughts, they are something we can all become masters of, one small, disobedient, intentional, courageous act of bravery at a time.

It's never too late to turn towards life and choose to ignore that voice of fear in your head—the one guiding you towards comfort, mediocrity, and smallness. I do not want to get to the end of it all begging my life like a toxic lover to just give me one last chance to love her, to cherish her properly, to give her all the attention she deserved, when time has all but run out.

Take me back, please! I'm sorry I took this body for granted. I promise I will cherish and savor every moment. Just please give me one more chance. To wear what I want and not care what others think. To look at the sky instead of my phone. To jump into puddles. To go out even when it's rainy and not give a shit if it ruins my hair. To touch the petals of flowers given to me on my birthday. To finally tell people the way I like to have sex so that I can actually enjoy it. To tell that person I love them. To laugh until it hurts and not care how I look or sound. To feel the sun on my face. To laugh at my fears and do whatever the fuck I want. To quit that job and travel like I always wanted to. To eat and not worry about how I will look the next day. To say how I feel instead of what I think people want to hear. To say "NO." To say "FUCK YES!" To dance more. To create more art. To live life as though life itself is a luxury which I can now see it was. I didn't even get to thank the people I love for the things they do. I didn't express myself enough. I never got to reach my potential. Take me back. Take me back so I can cherish you with the urgency and attention you deserve!

If you're reading this, it means that you're still alive. That it's *not* too late. That your life still belongs to you and there is time left to appreciate it. That there is time left, to start living deliciously.

Small doesn't suit you, anyway.

You were built for bigger things, and you fucking know it.

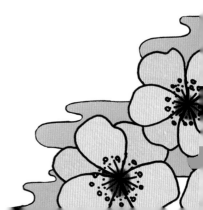

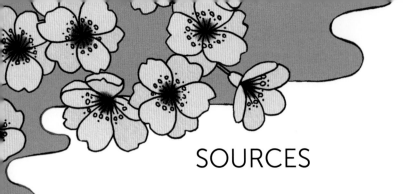

SOURCES

Bandura, Albert. "Towards a Psychology of Human Agency," *Perspectives on Psychological Science* 1 no. 2 (June 2006).

Berger, John. *Ways of Seeing* (New York: Penguin, 1972).

Brown, Brené. *Rising Strong: The Reckoning. The Rumble. The Revolution.* (New York: Vermilion, 2015).

Brown, Brené. *The Gifts of Imperfection. 10th Anniversary Edition* (New York: Vermilion, 2020).

Bryson, Kelly Bryson. *Don't Be Nice, Be Real: Balancing Passion for Self with Compassion for Others* (East Sussex, UK: Rudolph Steiner Press, 2002).

Cameron, Julia. *The Artist's Way: A Spiritual Path to Higher Creativity* (London, UK: Souvenir Press, 2020).

Clear, James. *Atomic Habits* (New York: Random House Business, 2018)

De Becker, Gavin. *The Gift of Fear: Survival Signs that Protect Us from Violence* (New York: Little, Brown, 1997).

Dillard, Annie. *The Writing Life* (New York: Harper Collins, 2013).

Doyle, Glennon. *Untamed: Stop Pleasing, Start Living* (New York: Vermilion, 2020).

Engeln, Renee. *Beauty Sick: How the Cultural Obsession with Appearance Hurts Girls and Women* (New York: Harper, 2017).

Freeman, Jo. "Trashing: The Dark Side of Sisterhood," originally published in *Ms*, April 1976.

Gilbert, Elizabeth. *Eat Pray Love* (New York: Viking Press, 2006).

Gottman, John and Silver, Nan. *The Seven Principles for Making Marriage Work* (London, UK: Orion Spring, 2023).

Hendricks, Gay. *The Big Leap: Conquer Your Hidden Fear and Take Life to the Next Level* (New York: Harper One, 2009).

hooks, bell. *All About Love: New Visions* (New York: Harper, 2000).

Housel, Morgan. *The Psychology of Money: Timeless Lessons on Wealth, Greed, and Happiness* (Hampshire, UK: Harriman House, 2020).

Keltner, Dacher. "What is Awe?" *Greater Good Magazine*, accessed 2024.

Kite, Lindsay and Lexie. *More Than a Body: Your Body Is an Instrument, Not an Ornament* (Eugene, OR: Harvest House, 2021).

Nin, Anaïs. *The Diary of Anaïs Nin,* vol. 3 (1939–1944) (New York: Houghton Mifflin, 2009)

Perez, Caroline Criado. *Invisible Women: Data Bias in a World Designed for Men* (London, UK: Chatto & Windus, 2019).

Odell, Jenny. *How to Do Nothing* (New York: Melville House Publishing, 2019).

Piff, P. K., Dietze, P., Feinburg, M., Stancato, D. M., and Keltner, D. "Awe, the Small Self, and Prosocial Behavior," Journal of Personality and Social Psychology 108(6), 2015.

Riess, Helen. *The Empathy Effect: Seven Neuroscience-Based Keys for Transforming the Way we Live, Love, Work, and Connect Across Differences* (Louisville, CO: Sounds True, 2018).

Singer, Michael. *The Untethered Soul: The Journey Beyond Yourself* (Oakland, CA: New Harbinger Publications, 2007).

Swart, Dr. Tara. *The Source: Open Your Mind, Change Your Life* (New York: Vermilion, 2019).

Tolle, Eckhart. *The Power of Now: A Guide to Spiritual Enlightenment* (20th Anniversary edition) (London, UK: Yellow Kite, 2001).

van der Kolk, Bessel. *The Body Keeps the Score: Mind, Brain, and Body in the Transformation of Trauma* (London, UK: Allen Lane, 2014).

Ware, Bronnie. *The Top Five Regrets of the Dying: A Life Transformed by the Dearly Departing* (London: Hay House UK, 2019).

Wolf, Naomi. *The Beauty Myth: How Images of Beauty Are Used Against Women* (London, UK: Chatto & Windus, 1990).

RESOURCES

Mindfulness: The Center for Mindfulness in Medicine, Health Care, and Society at the University of Massachusetts Medical School has published a useful report on members of the population who should not be encouraged to participate in mindfulness-based stress reduction: "Mindfulness-based Stress Reduction (MBSR): Standards of Practice" (edited and revised by Saki F. Santorelli), February 2014.

Suicide prevention: There are organizations that offer year-round support if you are struggling with mental health. These include The Samaritans, who can be contacted in the UK on 116 123; The National Suicide Prevention Lifeline, who can be contacted in the US at 1-800-271-8255; 9-8-8 Suicide Crisis, who can be contacted in Canada on 988; Lifeline, who can be contacted in Australia on 13 11 14 or in New Zealand on 0800 543 354.

For other organizations, www.befrienders.org is a helpful resource.

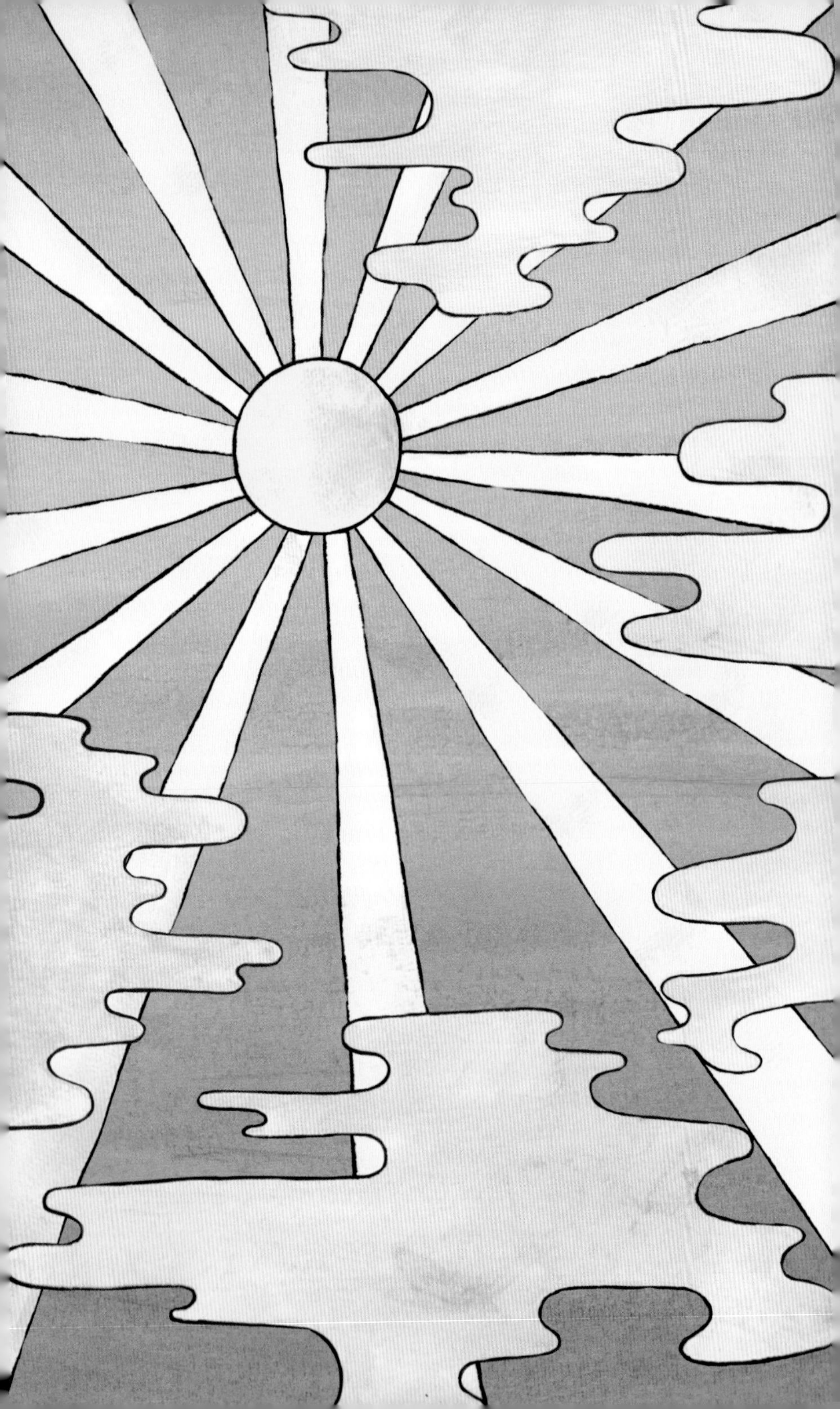

GRATITUDE

I am grateful to my editor Romilly, who has now worked across all three of my books, for coaching the best writing out of me. I've said this before, but you're so brilliant it's frightening. You encourage me to expand beyond what I think I am capable of and for that I am eternally grateful. Abi my book agent, for seeing something in me years ago that she believed needed to be shared with the world. You're the best cheerleader and I'm lucky to have you in my corner. Mel, for working with me to bring my vision for the layout and cover of this book to life. Pauline, for your feedback and suggestions to ensure this book was the best it could be. Those closest to me in my life, for the relentless encouragement, love, and support. To the universe, for guiding me through this entire process and revealing the next steps to me in the form of signs, songs, books, teachers, conversations, ideas; exactly when I needed them, no sooner or later. I feel as though we created this book together. Tokyo, I will love you forever. Thank you for providing the space I needed away from my life to slow down and allow the ideas that wanted to be manifested in this book the room to reveal themselves. The lovely baristas who served me coffee in the cafés where I sat writing. The music I listened to. The books I read. The ducks on my morning walks. The random pink flowers that grew in bushes, pavements, and gardens that I received as daily encouragement from the universe to keep writing the book. I wrote this book because I believe in the contagious effect of people who love their lives and that this joy, derived from authenticity, has the ability to impact the world. So I must thank every single wild, misunderstood, "cringey," authentic person that chooses to live a life on their own terms, in spite of the reactions it receives. You're forging the path for others to do the same. The world would not be delicious, but terribly fucking bland, without you.